Nursing Care

In

Dermatology

The complete Guide

ALEXANDRE CAREWELL

Table of Contents

Chapter 1: Introduction to Dermatology — 15
- Definition and importance of dermatology — 15
- A brief history of dermatology — 16
- Role and importance of the dermatology nurse — 17

Chapter 2: Anatomy and physiology of the skin — 19
- Skin structure — 19
- Functions and roles of the skin — 20
- Common skin diseases — 22

Chapter 3: Role of the dermatology nurse — 24
- Daily tasks and responsibilities — 24
- Interprofessional collaboration: working with dermatologists, surgeons and other specialists — 25
- Patient management and human relations — 27

Chapter 4: Common techniques and procedures — 30

- Skin samples: biopsies and cultures — 30
- Topical therapies: ointments, creams and gels — 32
- Wound management and suture care — 34

Chapter 5: Common dermatological conditions — 36

- Inflammatory skin diseases: eczema, psoriasis — 36
- Infectious conditions: herpes, warts — 38
- Tumour disorders: melanoma, carcinoma — 40
- Age- and sun-related skin diseases — 42

Chapter 6: Specific dermatological treatments — 45

- Phototherapy — 45
- Systemic therapies: corticosteroids, immunosuppressants — 46
- Biological therapies and new advances — 47

Chapter 7: Managing dermatological emergencies — 49

- Burns and traumatic injuries — 49
- Acute allergic reactions — 50
- Conditions requiring rapid intervention — 51

Chapter 8: Paediatric dermatology — 54

Special features of children's skin	54
Common ailments in children	55
Communication and special care for young patients	57

Chapter 9: Cosmetic and surgical dermatology — 60

Common cosmetic procedures	60
Surgical techniques in dermatology	62
Post-operative care and prevention of complications	64

Chapter 10: Challenges and ethics in dermatology — 66

Managing patients with chronic illnesses	66
Ethical issues relating to cosmetology	68
Continuity of care and psychological support	69

Chapter 11: Psychology and emotional support — 72

Psychological impact of skin disorders	72
A holistic approach to the patient: beyond the skin	73
Providing emotional support and tailored advice	75

Chapter 12: Diversity and specific skin care products — 77

- Ethnic differences and specific skincare requirements — 77
- Pigmentation disorders and specific concerns — 78
- Tackling diversity with sensitivity and skill — 80

Chapter 13: Technology in dermatology — 82

- The latest diagnostic tools — 82
- Telemedicine and remote consultations — 83
- Electronic records management and care coordination — 85

Chapter 14: Prevention and education — 87

- Raising awareness of the dangers of the sun and sun protection — 87
- Skin self-examination and early detection — 88
- Educating patients about daily skin care — 90

Chapter 15: Administrative and management aspects — 92

- Care coordination and appointment management — 92
- Financial aspects and insurance — 93

    Management of supplies, equipment and medicines   95

Chapter 16: Dermatology and systemic pathologies   97

    Skin manifestations of internal diseases   97

    The nurse and autoimmune diseases with dermatological manifestations   98

    Collaboration with other specialities for integrated monitoring   100

Chapter 17: Skin infections and tropical diseases   102

    Recognition of common and rare infections   102

    An approach to skin diseases linked to travel and geography   103

    Prevention and advice for travellers   105

Chapter 18: Dermatology in specific contexts   107

    Dermatology in hospital versus private practice   107

    Dermatology in rural versus urban areas   109

    Dermatological care in emergency or disaster situations   110

Chapter 19: Legal aspects of dermatology   113

- Informed consent and invasive procedures — 113
- Managing complications and medical errors — 115
- Patients' rights and professional responsibilities — 116

Chapter 20: Dermatology and vulnerable populations — 119

- Dermatological care for the elderly — 119
- Dermatology and immunocompromised patients — 120
- Skin care for patients at the end of life — 122

Chapter 21: Pain and symptom management — 125

- Dealing with chronic pain associated with skin disorders — 125
- Palliative care in dermatology — 126
- Non-pharmacological strategies for managing pain and pruritus — 128

Chapter 22: Psychodermatological aspects — 131

- The interface between psychology and dermatology — 131
- Management of conditions such as psychogenic pruritus and trichotillomania — 132

The role of the nurse in the management of psychodermatological disorders	134

Chapter 23: Dermatology and global health — 136

The impact of diet and lifestyle on the skin	136
Physical activity, stress and skin	137
Integrating dermatology into a holistic approach to health	139

Chapter 24: Allergies and skin tests — 141

Fundamentals of skin allergy testing	141
Interpreting and communicating results	142
Care and monitoring of allergy sufferers	144

Chapter 25: Dermatology and sexuality — 147

STIs and skin manifestations	147
Education, prevention and advice	148
Discussing sexuality in dermatology consultations	150

Chapter 26: Nail and hair diseases — 152

Recognition of common ailments	152
Specific nursing interventions and care	153

- Practical advice for patients — 155

Chapter 27: New treatments and therapies — 158

- Exploring recent advances — 158
- Gene and targeted therapies — 160
- The future of biotechnology in dermatology — 161

Chapter 28: Hospital hygiene and infection prevention — 163

- The importance of sterilisation and disinfection in dermatology — 163
- Risk management and prevention of nosocomial infections — 164
- The role of the nurse in implementing hygiene protocols — 166

Chapter 29: Dermatology and aesthetics — 169

- The evolution of medical aesthetics — 169
- The ethical implications of aesthetics in dermatology — 171
- The role of the nurse in aesthetic procedures — 172

Chapter 30: Development and career in dermatology — 175

- Specialisation opportunities — 175
- Ongoing training and skills updating — 176

    The future of dermatology: new 178
    advances and technologies

Chapter 31: Conclusion and additional 181
resources

    Resources to expand your knowledge 181

    Professional networks and associations 184

    Personal and professional development 186
    in dermatology

« Dermatology: medical speciality devoted to the prevention, diagnosis and treatment of diseases of the skin, hair, nails and mucous membranes. »

Chapter 1:
INTRODUCTION TO DERMATOLOGY

Definition and importance dermatology

Dermatology, at the crossroads of art and science, is the medical branch specialising in the health and diseases of the skin, hair, nails and mucous membranes. But to reduce dermatology to a simple observation of the surface would be to underestimate it. For the skin, that fascinating organ, is the mirror of our body, often reflecting signs of internal disorders or systemic disturbances. From teenage acne to the cutaneous signs of lupus, dermatology encompasses a surprisingly broad spectrum of conditions and pathologies.

Yet the importance of dermatology goes far beyond its technical definition. In a society where appearance and self-esteem are intrinsically linked, healthy skin has profound implications for an individual's confidence and psychological well-being. Who hasn't felt that little dip in morale when faced with an unexpected rash or unwanted mark? That's where dermatology comes in, not only as a curative science, but also as a preventative one, enabling everyone to feel good about themselves, literally and figuratively.

What's more, as medical technology continues to evolve rapidly, dermatology is constantly adapting and innovating. It is at the cutting edge of discoveries, whether in laser treatments, gene therapies or cosmetic procedures. But at the heart of this speciality remains a fundamental objective: to understand and treat the individual as a whole, taking into account the complex interaction between skin, mind and body.

It's a discipline that demands special sensitivity from its practitioners, because every mark and every scar has a story to tell. And every patient comes with the hope of finding answers, solutions and sometimes, a transformation. Dermatology is not just about skin; it goes to the very essence of who we are, how we interact with the world and how the world sees us.

A brief history of dermatology

The history of dermatology, like that of medicine in general, is long and complex, marked by discoveries, errors, advances and innovations. Interest in the skin and its ailments dates back to antiquity, with medical references found in ancient Egyptian, Greek, Roman, Chinese and Indian texts.

In ancient Egypt, the skin was already the focus of attention, and ointments and salves were developed to treat a variety of skin conditions. Hippocrates, the father of modern medicine, listed conditions such as urticaria, scabies and other skin diseases.

However, it was during the Middle Ages in Europe that the foundations of modern dermatology began to take shape. Skin diseases, often associated with superstition and religious beliefs, were treated by barber-surgeons rather than physicians. Leprosy, in particular, had a profound impact on the perception and treatment of skin disorders.

The real turning point for dermatology came in the 19th century. With the advent of the scientific method and improved diagnostic tools, the field experienced an explosion of knowledge. In France, Jean-Louis Alibert and Ferdinand Rayer were pioneers, laying the foundations of clinical dermatology. They were followed by others across

Europe, who systematically classified and documented various skin diseases.

The 20th century saw the advent of the first effective therapies for many skin conditions, with the discovery of antibiotics, the advent of dermatological surgery and the development of the first laser treatments. The second half of the century was marked by an unprecedented advance in our understanding of the molecular and genetic mechanisms underlying skin diseases.

Today, dermatology is at the confluence of traditional science and technological innovation. With advances in molecular biology, genomics, and laser technology, dermatology is better equipped than ever to meet patients' needs, offering solutions for conditions once considered incurable. In this way, this brief history is a testament to the resilience and continued evolution of a field focused on health, wellbeing and, inevitably, our human identity.

Role and importance of the dermatology nurse

The dermatology nurse is much more than a simple assistant to the dermatologist. They play a central role in patient care, combining technical skills with human qualities.

Firstly, the dermatology nurse is often the first point of contact for the patient. He or she takes the patient's medical history, assesses the severity of symptoms and guides the patient towards the most appropriate course of treatment. Through this initial contact, they play an essential role in reassuring patients, who are often worried or embarrassed by skin symptoms.

Nurses also carry out a number of technical procedures: preparing and assisting with minor surgical procedures, applying complex dressings, administering topical or systemic treatments, and providing therapeutic education to teach patients how to manage their illness on a day-to-day basis.

But beyond these technical skills, the dermatology nurse plays a vital role in the psychological care of patients. Skin conditions, which are visible and sometimes stigmatising, can have a profound impact on self-esteem and quality of life. The nurse is there to listen, advise and support the patient throughout the treatment process, often demonstrating empathy and patience.

Patient education is also at the heart of the profession. Whether it's the correct application of a treatment, sun protection or the early detection of signs of complications, the nurse is a health educator, arming patients with the knowledge they need to take control of their health.

With the rapid evolution of medicine and technology, the dermatology nurse is also constantly training, keeping abreast of the latest advances to provide the best possible care.

The dermatology nurse is a central pillar of the medical team. Through their close relationship with patients, their technical skills and their role as educators, they make an invaluable contribution to the well-being of patients and the quality of dermatology care. His or her reassuring presence and expertise are essential in providing comprehensive, humane care for every individual he or she encounters.

Chapter 2:
SKIN ANATOMY AND PHYSIOLOGY

Skin structure

The skin, the largest external organ of the human body, is much more than just a protective envelope. Its complex structure enables it to perform a wide range of functions, including protection from external aggressors, thermal regulation and sensation. To understand these functions, it is essential to look at its multi-layered structure and the different cells that make it up.

1. The epidermis: This is the superficial layer of the skin, in direct contact with the environment. It is mainly made up of keratinocytes, cells that produce keratin, a protein that gives the skin its protective properties. The epidermis is subdivided into several layers, from the basal layer, where new keratinocytes are constantly produced, to the stratum corneum, where the cells are completely keratinised and eventually shed. This layer also includes melanocytes, responsible for the production of melanin (skin pigment), and Langerhans cells, key players in the cutaneous immune response.

2. The dermis: Located just below the epidermis, the dermis is a thick, dense layer composed mainly of collagen and elastin fibres, which give the skin its strength and elasticity. It also contains the skin's appendages, such as the sebaceous glands, sweat glands and hair follicles. The dermis is rich in blood vessels, lymphatics and nerves, which enable it to provide the skin with nutrition, evacuate waste products and transmit sensations.

3. The hypodermis: This is the deepest layer, mainly composed of adipose tissue. The hypodermis acts as a thermal insulator, an energy reserve and plays a role in protection against physical shocks. It also provides the link between the skin and underlying tissues such as muscles and bones.

Beyond these three main layers, the skin is packed with sensory receptors, enabling it to perceive a variety of stimuli, such as temperature, pressure or pain. These receptors, combined with a dense nervous network, make the skin a sensory organ in its own right, in constant interaction with its environment.

The structure of the skin reflects its complexity and adaptability. This organ, both barrier and interface, plays a crucial role in protection, regulation and perception, while constantly adapting to the needs and aggressions of everyday life.

Functions and roles of the skin

The skin, often described as the body's envelope, fulfils a multitude of vital functions that go far beyond its simple outward appearance. It is a reflection of our health and well-being, and plays a key role in a number of physiological processes. To fully appreciate its importance, let's explore the main functions and roles of this remarkable organ.

1. Protection:
- **Physical barrier:** The horny layer of the epidermis, made up of keratinised cells, provides a first line of defence against mechanical, chemical and microbial aggression.
- **Immune barrier:** Langerhans cells in the epidermis are immune sentinels that detect and react to pathogens.

UV protection: By producing melanin, melanocytes protect the skin against the harmful effects of ultraviolet rays.

2. Thermal control :

Sweat: The sweat glands produce sweat, which evaporates to cool the surface of the skin and help regulate body temperature.

Vasodilation and vasoconstriction: The blood vessels in the skin can dilate or contract to release or retain heat.

3. Sensation :

Thanks to a dense network of nerve receptors, the skin is sensitive to various stimuli such as temperature, pressure, pain and touch. This sensory perception connects us to our environment and contributes to our experience of the world.

4. Synthesis and secretion :

Vitamin D: Under the effect of UVB rays, the skin synthesises vitamin D, which is essential for bone health.

Sebum: The sebaceous glands produce sebum, an oily substance that lubricates and waterproofs the skin.

5. Absorption :

The skin can absorb certain drugs, chemicals and substances, hence the importance of proper skin care and the popularity of medicated patches.

6. Energy reserves :

The hypodermis, made up of adipose tissue, serves as an energy reserve for the body. This layer stores lipids, providing a source of energy when needed.

7. Aesthetics and communication :

The skin reflects our general state of health, our emotions (such as blushing) and contributes to our visual identity. It plays a role in social interaction and self-perception.

The skin is a versatile and dynamic organ that plays an essential role in many vital functions. Its ability to interact with the environment, protect the body and participate in various physiological functions is testament to its importance to our overall well-being.

Common skin diseases

As the interface between our body and the environment, the skin is susceptible to a myriad of disorders. These disorders can result from genetic, environmental, infectious or immune factors, or from allergic reactions. Here is an overview of some of the most common skin diseases:

1. Acne :
Characterised by eruptions of pimples, blackheads and cysts, acne is often due to an overproduction of sebum associated with an obstruction of the pilosebaceous follicles.

2. Eczema (or atopic dermatitis):
This is a chronic inflammatory skin condition causing itching, redness and scaling. It may be due to genetic, allergic or environmental factors.

3. Psoriasis :
This is a chronic inflammatory skin disease characterised by red patches covered with whitish scales. It may be associated with genetic or immune factors.

4. Hives:
Featuring red, itchy patches, hives can be triggered by many factors, including allergens, infections, medication or stress.

5. Skin mycoses :
Caused by fungi, these infections can affect different parts of the body, including the feet (athlete's foot), the nails, or the body in general. They appear as red, scaly patches and can be accompanied by itching.

6. Vitiligo :
This autoimmune condition is manifested by the disappearance of pigmentation in certain areas of the skin, giving colourless white patches.

7. Herpes :
Caused by the herpes simplex virus, this infection manifests as outbreaks of painful blisters, usually around the mouth or genitals.

8. Shingles :
This is a reactivation of the varicella-zoster virus, usually associated with painful rashes and blisters along a nerve.

9. Rosacea :
It is characterised by redness, visible small vessels, pustules and papules, generally on the face.

10. Warts :
Caused by the human papillomavirus (HPV), these small growths can appear on any part of the body.

11. Melanoma :
This is the most aggressive form of skin cancer, often associated with excessive sun exposure or a family history.

It is essential to note that in the event of any skin anomaly or persistent symptoms, it is advisable to consult a dermatologist. Early detection and appropriate treatment are crucial for many of these conditions.

Chapter 3:
THE ROLE OF THE NURSE IN DERMATOLOGY

Daily tasks and responsibilities

Dermatology nurses play a crucial role in the care of patients suffering from skin diseases. In addition to their general nursing duties, they have specific responsibilities linked to this speciality. Here is a detailed overview of their day-to-day duties and responsibilities:

1. Clinical assessment :
    - Carry out an initial examination of the patient's skin, noting the areas affected and the type and extent of lesions.
    - Regular monitoring to assess the progress of the disease and the effectiveness of treatment.
2. Treatment administration :
    - Apply creams, lotions or topical medication.
    - Assisting the dermatologist with procedures such as biopsies, cryotherapy or phototherapy.
    - Administer medication orally, intravenously or subcutaneously, as prescribed.
3. Patient education :
    - Teaching patients about good skin hygiene practices.
    - Explain treatments, their potential side effects and how to manage them.
    - Advice on prevention, particularly sun protection.
4. Psychological support :
    - Offer emotional support, as some skin conditions can affect confidence and self-esteem.
    - Refer, if necessary, to specialist resources such as support groups or psychologists.
5. Care coordination :

Working closely with the dermatologist, but also with other health professionals (allergists, nutritionists, plastic surgeons, etc.).

Organising and scheduling appointments for complementary examinations or surgical procedures.

6. Keeping medical records :

Accurately document all the care provided, observations and changes in the patient's skin condition.

Updating medical records after each consultation or treatment.

7. Maintaining professional skills :

Regularly attend training courses and seminars to keep up to date with the latest advances in dermatology.

Working with peers to share knowledge and experience.

8. Management of equipment and hygiene :

Ensuring the cleanliness and sterilisation of the instruments and equipment used.

Ensure that medical supplies are well stocked.

Dermatology nurses play an essential role in the care of patients suffering from skin disorders. They combine clinical skills, listening skills and teaching skills to provide holistic, tailored care.

Interprofessional collaboration: working with dermatologists, surgeons and other specialists

Modern medicine, particularly in a field as vast and interconnected as dermatology, relies on close collaboration between different healthcare professionals. Dermatology nurses do not work in silos, but as part of a multidisciplinary team. Let's take a look at how this collaboration works, and why it's essential for optimal patient care.

1. With dermatologists :
    - **Regular communication:** The nurse informs the dermatologist of the patient's condition, concerns and reactions to treatment.
    - **Assistance during procedures:** During biopsies, cryotherapy or other interventions, the nurse prepares the equipment, assists the dermatologist and ensures the patient's comfort.
    - **Referral:** Because of their close relationship with the patient, nurses can identify specific needs and suggest an in-depth consultation with the dermatologist.
2. With plastic and reconstructive surgeons:
    - **Patient transfers: In the** case of lesions requiring surgery (such as melanoma), the nurse coordinates the transfer of the patient to the surgeon.
    - **Pre-operative preparation:** The nurse prepares the patient for surgery, providing information on the procedure, risks and post-operative care.
    - **Post-operative follow-up:** After the operation, the nurse is often the first point of contact for wound care, pain management and monitoring any complications.
3. With other specialists:
    - **Allergists:** For cases of eczema, urticaria or other allergic reactions, the nurse can work with the allergist to identify allergens and adjust treatments.
    - **Nutritionists:** Some skin problems can be linked to diet. The nurse can refer the patient to a nutritionist for specific dietary advice.
    - **Rheumatologists: In the case of** psoriasis, there is a risk of developing psoriatic arthritis. Collaboration between the nurse, the dermatologist and the rheumatologist is crucial to comprehensive care.

Psychologists: Skin diseases can have a major psychological impact. The nurse may suggest a psychological consultation to help the patient manage the stress, anxiety or depression associated with their skin condition.

4. Collaboration with other nurses :

Ongoing training, exchanges of experience and coordination of care between specialist nurses are essential to ensure consistent, high-quality care.

Interprofessional collaboration enables holistic patient care. Each professional contributes his or her expertise, ensuring that all aspects of the patient's health are taken into account. For the dermatology nurse, this collaboration is essential to ensure optimal, individualised care.

Patient management and human relations

Patient management in dermatology goes far beyond the simple treatment of skin conditions. It involves a deep understanding of patients' emotional, psychological and social needs. Human relationships are at the heart of this process. Let's look at how the dermatology nurse manages these essential aspects of care.

1. Establishing trust :

   Active listening: The nurse must pay attention to the patient's concerns, ask open-ended questions and validate the patient's feelings.

   Empathy: Understanding and sharing the patient's feelings strengthens the therapeutic bond.

2. Education and communication :

   Clear information: Nurses must explain diagnoses, treatments and procedures in an understandable way, avoiding over-complex medical jargon.

- **Encouraging dialogue:** Patients should feel comfortable asking questions, expressing concerns or seeking clarification.

3. Managing anxiety and stress :
   - **Emotional support:** Skin conditions can affect self-esteem. The nurse must offer emotional support, reassure the patient and, if necessary, recommend psychological help.
   - **Relaxation techniques:** In some cases, nurses may teach breathing or relaxation techniques to help manage anxiety linked to procedures or treatments.

4. Confidentiality :
   - **Respect for privacy:** Nurses must always ensure the confidentiality of patients' medical and personal information.
   - **One-to-one discussion:** Offering a private space to discuss sensitive or intimate concerns.

5. Cultural sensitivity :
   - **Understanding differences:** Cultural beliefs, values and practices can influence the way people perceive and manage their illness. Nurses must be aware of and respect these differences.
   - **Interpreters and resources:** If necessary, use interpreters or other resources to ensure clear and effective communication.

6. Working with family and friends :
   - **Integration into the care process:** Involving the family can strengthen emotional support and help manage treatments at home.
   - **Education:** Teaching family and friends about basic care, recognising symptoms and when to seek help.

7. Expectation management :
   - **Honesty:** Informing patients of what they can reasonably expect from treatment, while avoiding raising false hopes.

Regular feedback: keeping patients informed of changes in their condition and adjusting expectations accordingly.

Managing patients in dermatology requires a patient-centred approach, where clinical skills are combined with genuine humanity. The nurse, through his or her proximity and regular contact with the patient, plays a central role in creating this relationship of trust and mutual respect.

Chapter 4:
TECHNIQUES AND STANDARD PROCEDURES

Skin samples : biopsies and cultures

Skin samples, such as biopsies and cultures, are common procedures in dermatology to aid in the diagnosis and treatment of skin conditions. They are essential for understanding the exact nature of the lesion or infection and for guiding management. Nurses play a crucial role in preparing, carrying out and monitoring these procedures.

1. Understanding the reasons :
    - **Biopsy:** This tissue sample is taken to examine the cells under a microscope, making it possible to diagnose various conditions, such as skin cancer or inflammation.
    - **Culture:** This is used to identify infectious agents, such as bacteria or fungi, by growing them in the laboratory.
2. Preparing the patient :
    - **Information:** The nurse must explain the procedure, its reasons and its benefits to the patient.
    - **Informed consent:** Ensure that the patient understands the implications and obtain written consent.
    - **Preparing the area:** Clean and disinfect the area concerned.
3. Taking the sample :
    - Biopsy :
        - **Common types :** There are different types of biopsy (puncture, incisional, excisional) depending on the size and nature of the lesion.

Anaesthesia: A local anaesthetic is often administered to reduce discomfort.
   Technique: The nurse, in collaboration with the dermatologist, takes a tissue sample using a sharp instrument.
   Culture :
   Sampling: A sample is taken, often using a swab, from an area suspected of being infected.
   Transfer: The sample is placed in an appropriate culture medium and sent to the laboratory for analysis.
4. Post-procedure care :
   Instructions: Inform the patient about wound care, monitoring for signs of infection and the importance of keeping the area clean and dry.
   Follow-up: Schedule an appointment to remove the stitches, if necessary, and discuss the results.
   Pain management: Advise the patient on pain management, including the use of over-the-counter analgesics or the prescription of medication, if necessary.
5. Communication of results :
   Biopsy results: The results can help confirm a diagnosis, determine the stage of a disease or guide treatment.
   Culture results: These identify the infectious agent and, often, its sensitivity to antimicrobials.
6. The role of the nurse :
   Reassurance: The nurse offers emotional support, especially if the patient is anxious or worried about the results.
   Coordination: The nurse works with the laboratory and the dermatologist to ensure that samples are processed correctly and that results are communicated in good time.

Skin samples are essential diagnostic tools in dermatology. Thanks to their expertise, nurses play a central role in the success of these procedures, guaranteeing patient safety, comfort and information throughout the process.

Topical therapies : ointments, creams and gels

In the vast field of dermatology, topical therapies, particularly ointments, creams and gels, play a key role. They provide direct treatment for skin conditions and offer a variety of therapeutic options. Nurses, at the heart of patient care, play an essential role in the application, education and monitoring of these treatments.

1. Understanding the basics :
    Formulations :
    - **Ointments:** oil-based preparations, often occlusive, ideal for very dry skin.
    - **Creams:** water-in-oil or oil-in-water emulsions, suitable for most skin types.
    - **Gels:** water-based, lightweight and often used for oily areas or conditions such as acne.

    Active ingredients: Varies depending on the condition being treated, which may include corticosteroids, antimicrobials, antifungals, keratolytic agents, among others.

2. Correct application :
    - **Cleaning:** Start by gently cleansing the affected area.
    - **Quantity:** Use the prescribed quantity, generally a thin coat.
    - **Technique:** Apply gently, without rubbing excessively. Some treatments require a light massage.

3. Patient education :

Frequency: Inform the patient about the frequency of application.

Side effects: Discuss potential side effects and how to recognise them.

Storage: Advise on how to store the product to ensure it remains effective.

Interactions: Talk about other products or medicines that could interact with topical treatment.

4. Managing side effects :

Irritation: Some products may cause redness or itching. It is essential to assess the severity and adjust treatment if necessary.

Skin atrophy: Topical corticosteroids, when used long-term, can cause thinning of the skin. Regular monitoring is essential.

Allergic reactions: Recognising the signs of an allergic reaction and advising the patient on the steps to take.

5. The importance of adhesion :

Regularity: Emphasise the importance of regular application to maximise benefits.

Duration: Some treatments require prolonged use to see results, while others are shorter.

6. Role of the nurse :

Demonstration: Show the patient the correct application technique.

Evaluation: Regularly review the condition of the patient's skin to ensure the treatment is effective.

Feedback: Encourage patients to share their experiences and adjust treatment if necessary.

Topical therapies are a mainstay of dermatological treatment. Through their practical and educational approach, nurses ensure that patients benefit fully from these treatments, guaranteeing that they are used safely, effectively and in a way that is adapted to each individual case.

Wound management and suture care

Care of wounds and sutures is an essential part of dermatology, particularly after surgery or biopsies. The aim of this care is to promote optimal healing, prevent infection and minimise scarring. Nurses, with their skills and know-how, are at the forefront of ensuring the quality of this care and educating patients about it.

1. Initial wound assessment :
    - **Depth and extent:** Identify the severity of the wound to choose the best treatment protocol.
    - **Signs of infection:** Look for redness, heat, swelling, pus or excessive pain.
    - **Type of suture:** Sutures can be absorbable or non-absorbable, superficial or deep.
2. Cleaning and disinfection :
    - **Physiological saline:** This is often used to gently clean the wound.
    - **Antiseptics:** Application of agents such as chlorhexidine or povidone-iodine to disinfect.
3. Suture care :
    - **Protection:** Use of sterile dressings to protect the wound from contaminants.
    - **Avoidance:** It is advisable not to wet the sutured area for the first 24 to 48 hours.
    - **Observation:** Watch for signs of tension or loosening of the sutures.
4. Changing dressings :
    - **Frequency:** Depending on the doctor's recommendations, some dressings need to be changed regularly.

Technique: Remove carefully to avoid aggravating the wound or pulling on the sutures.
5. Scar prevention :
Moisturising: Applying moisturising agents can help reduce scarring.
Sun protection: Healed wounds can be sensitive to the sun, so it's important to use sunscreen to avoid hyperpigmentation.
6. Patient education :
Post-operative instructions: Provide clear instructions on care at home, recognising complications and when to seek advice.
Mobilisation: Advise the patient on activities to avoid in order to prevent tension on the wound.
7. Removal of sutures :
Timing: Removal is generally carried out according to a precise timetable, depending on the location and nature of the wound.
Technique: Use of sterile forceps and scissors, taking care to minimise discomfort.
8. Role of the nurse :
Communication: reassuring the patient, explaining each stage of care and answering any questions.
Monitoring: Identify and treat any complications rapidly.
Coordination: Work with the dermatologist or surgeon to ensure appropriate follow-up.

Effective wound management and suture care are crucial to ensuring uncomplicated healing. Nurses, through their training and experience, ensure that every patient receives quality care, while being a pillar of information and support throughout the healing process.

Chapter 5:
COMMON DERMATOLOGICAL CONDITIONS

Inflammatory skin diseases : eczema, psoriasis

Inflammatory dermatoses, including eczema and psoriasis, are common skin conditions affecting many people around the world. Characterised by inflammation and skin lesions, they can cause significant discomfort and have an impact on patients' quality of life. The dermatology nurse is at the heart of the management, education and support of patients with these conditions.

1. Eczema (atopic dermatitis) :
    Features :
        - Redness, pruritus, dry patches.
        - Can be triggered by allergens, irritants or environmental factors.
    Treatments :
        - **Moisturising:** Applying creams and ointments to restore the skin barrier.
        - **Topical corticosteroids:** To reduce inflammation.
        - **Antihistamines:** To control itching.
        - **Systemic treatments:** In severe or refractory cases.
    Role of the nurse :
        - **Education:** Educating the patient about potential triggers and how to minimise flare-ups.
        - **Application:** Demonstrate the correct way to apply medicines.

Monitoring: Regularly assess the condition of the skin and the effectiveness of the treatment.

2. Psoriasis :

Features :
Thick, red patches with silvery scales.
May be associated with joint pain in the case of arthropathic psoriasis.
Treatments :
Topical treatments: Corticosteroids, vitamin D derivatives, tazarotene.
Phototherapy: Use of UVB light to reduce inflammation.
Systemic treatments: Drugs such as methotrexate or cyclosporine.
Biological treatments: Injections that target specific parts of the immune system.
Role of the nurse :
Education: Informing the patient about the chronic nature of the disease and treatment options.
Monitoring: Assessing the side effects of treatments and adjusting dosages.
Support: Providing emotional support in the face of the psychosocial challenges associated with psoriasis.

3. Common factors :

Stress: Both conditions can be exacerbated by stress, so it's crucial to recognise its impact and suggest strategies for managing it.
Psychosocial aspect: The impact on self-esteem, anxiety and depression must be taken into account in treatment.
Links with other specialities: Sometimes it is necessary to collaborate with other health professionals, such as rheumatologists for arthropathic psoriasis.

4. The role of the nurse :
- **Communication:** Establishing a relationship of trust with the patient, responding to questions and concerns.
- **Care management:** coordinating with the dermatologist for an individualised care plan.
- **Research:** Keeping abreast of the latest advances and treatments available.

Inflammatory dermatoses, despite their prevalence, require tailored and nuanced management. Nurses play an essential role in providing quality care, education and essential support to patients, helping them to manage their condition effectively and improve their quality of life.

Infectious diseases : herpes, warts

Infectious skin conditions, such as herpes and warts, are caused by viruses and can affect many people at different stages of their lives. Although these infections are generally benign, they can cause discomfort and aesthetic concerns. Dermatology nurses play a vital role in diagnosing, treating and educating patients about these conditions.

1. Herpes :
- Features :
  - Painful, itchy vesicles, usually grouped together, often preceded by tingling or burning sensations.
  - May affect the mouth (herpes labialis) or genitals (genital herpes).
- Treatments :
  - **Antivirals:** Drugs such as acyclovir, valacyclovir and famciclovir to reduce the duration and severity of outbreaks.

Topical treatments: To relieve pain or associated pruritus.

Role of the nurse :

Education: Inform patients about the means of transmission, prevention methods and the need to avoid contact during outbreaks.

Support: Understanding the psychosocial distress associated with the diagnosis and offering appropriate support.

Monitoring: Monitoring of symptoms and adjustment of treatment if necessary.

2. Warts :

Features :

Rough growths caused by the human papillomavirus (HPV).

Can appear on the hands, feet and other parts of the body.

Treatments :

Cryotherapy: Use of liquid nitrogen to freeze the wart.

Topical treatments: Preparations based on salicylic acid or other ingredients to erode the wart.

Minor therapies: such as curettage, electrocoagulation or laser.

Role of the nurse :

Education: Explaining prevention methods and home care to patients.

Application: Demonstrate the correct way to apply topical treatments.

Follow-up: to ensure that warts respond well to treatment and to detect any complications.

3. Prevention :

Herpes: Use condoms, avoid direct contact during outbreaks, prophylactic antivirals for high-risk individuals.

- **Warts:** Do not touch or scratch warts, use shoes in public areas (such as gym showers), avoid sharing personal items.
4. The role of the nurse :
    - **Communication:** Establishing an open dialogue with the patient, clarifying myths and misconceptions.
    - **Care management:** coordinating with the dermatologist to ensure that the patient receives the most appropriate treatment.
    - **Update:** Keep up to date with the latest developments in treatment and prevention.

Although herpes and warts are common, their impact on patients' well-being can be significant. The dermatology nurse's proximity to the patient, expertise and teaching skills are essential in providing comprehensive, reassuring care.

Tumour disorders : melanoma, carcinoma

Skin tumours, including entities such as melanoma and carcinoma, are major pathologies in dermatology. These tumours, whether benign or malignant, require special attention, early detection and appropriate treatment. Dermatology nurses play a crucial role in supporting patients, from initial detection through to post-treatment follow-up.

1. Melanoma :
    - Features :
        - Malignant melanocytic cell cancer.
        - Often appears as a new pigmented lesion or an existing mole that changes appearance.
        - Risk factors include excessive sun exposure, family history and fair skin.

Treatments :
> **Surgical excision:** removal of the tumour and a margin of healthy tissue.
> **Targeted therapies and immunotherapy:** For advanced or metastatic melanoma.

Role of the nurse :
> **Education:** Raising awareness of the importance of skin self-examination and regular dermatological check-ups.
> **Support:** Offering emotional support in the face of diagnosis and during treatment.
> **Monitoring:** Post-operative scar monitoring, early detection of recurrence.

2. Carcinomas :

Features :

The most common are basal cell carcinoma (BCC) and squamous cell carcinoma (SCC).

Often appear on sun-exposed areas such as the face, ears and hands.

They may appear as nodules, red patches or ulcers that do not heal.

Treatments :

Surgical excision: removal of the tumour with a safety margin.

Cryosurgery, electrosurgery: For shallower lesions.

Topical therapies and phototherapy: In certain early or superficial cases.

Role of the nurse :

Education: Informing people about the risks associated with exposure to the sun and the importance of sun protection.

Support: Assisting patients during operations and post-operative care.

Monitoring: Ensuring that treated lesions heal and detecting any new lesions.

3. Prevention :
- **Sun protection:** Encourage regular use of sun creams, wear protective clothing, and avoid direct exposure to the sun during peak hours.
- **Screening:** Promote regular dermatological consultations, particularly for high-risk individuals.

4. The role of the nurse :
- **Communication:** Establishing a relationship of trust, clearly explaining diagnoses, treatments and expected outcomes.
- **Care management:** coordinating with the multidisciplinary team, including dermatologists, oncologists and surgeons.
- **Career development:** Keeping up to date with advances in treatment and surgical techniques.

Because of their potentially serious nature, skin tumours require a rigorous and empathetic approach. Dermatology nurses play a central role in patient care, guaranteeing optimum quality of care, combining technical expertise with human support.

Age- and sun-related skin diseases

With ageing and repeated exposure to the sun, the skin undergoes significant changes, giving rise to various dermatoses. Some of these conditions are benign, but can have an aesthetic impact, while others can present a health risk. Dermatology nurses play a central role in helping patients to understand, prevent and treat these conditions.

1. Actinic keratoses :
- Features :
  - Rough, thickened lesions caused by years of sun exposure.

Exposed surfaces such as the face, hands and scalp.
Treatments :
Cryosurgery: freezing of lesions.
Topical therapies: Chemical agents to eliminate abnormal cells.
Phototherapy: Use of light to treat lesions.
Role of the nurse :
Education: Raising awareness of the dangers of exposure to the sun.
Monitoring: Follow-up of lesions to detect any progression to carcinoma.

2. Sun spots (age spots) :
Features :
Flat, brown patches, usually on the face, hands and arms.
Resulting from cumulative sun exposure.
Treatments :
Laser therapies : To lighten or eliminate spots.
Chemical peels: Use of acids to exfoliate the skin.
Microdermabrasion: Mechanical exfoliation of the skin's surface.
Role of the nurse :
Tip: Offer solutions to prevent the appearance of new spots.
Support: Helping patients to understand and manage the aesthetic implications.

3. Solar elastosis :
Features :
Thick, yellow skin with deep wrinkles.
Resulting from the degradation of elastic fibres due to exposure to the sun.
Treatments :
Moisturising: creams and lotions to improve skin texture.

- **Aesthetic treatments:** To improve the appearance of the skin.
- Role of the nurse :
- **Education:** Sun prevention and protection.
- **Guidance:** Helping patients choose treatments suited to their condition.

4. Prevention :
   - **Sun protection:** Encourage the use of broad-spectrum sun creams, hats and long clothing.
   - **Regular check-ups:** Promote self-examination of the skin and dermatological consultations to detect early changes.

5. The role of the nurse :
   - **Communication:** Raising patients' awareness of the consequences of sun exposure and the benefits of adequate protection.
   - **Referral:** Directing patients to appropriate resources, whether for treatment or prevention.

Dermatoses linked to age and the sun can, in many cases, be prevented or reduced. The dermatology nurse, thanks to his or her in-depth knowledge and proximity to patients, is essential in providing holistic care, from prevention to therapy, while taking into account the patient's overall well-being.

Chapter 6:
SPECIFIC TREATMENTS IN DERMATOLOGY

Phototherapy

Phototherapy, as fascinating as it sounds, is a therapeutic approach that has come about through the fusion of science and light. It is based on the use of specific wavelengths of light to treat a range of dermatological conditions, with psoriasis and atopic eczema topping the list.

The concept behind phototherapy is simple: by exposing the skin to controlled doses of light, we can induce biological changes at cellular level that are beneficial in the treatment of certain skin conditions. However, not just any light will do. UVB light, for example, is the most commonly used because of its ability to slow the growth of skin cells, which is essential for treating conditions such as psoriasis where the skin renews itself too quickly.

But of course, as with any treatment, there are nuances. The intensity, duration and frequency of exposure must be carefully calibrated, not only to maximise effectiveness, but also to minimise the associated risks, such as burns or, in the long term, an increased risk of skin cancer.

Nurses play a key role in phototherapy. They guide patients through the process, ensuring that they wear adequate protection for the eyes and parts of the body that do not require treatment. They also closely monitor the skin's reaction to the light, adjusting the dose if necessary.

The beauty of phototherapy lies in its ability to offer an alternative or complement to topical and systemic treatments, often without the side effects associated with the latter. Many patients find significant relief with this method, renewing their self-confidence and comfort in their own skin.

So the next time you hear about phototherapy, think of this harmonious dance between light and skin, orchestrated by dedicated professionals to restore balance and health to the skin. It's a brilliant reminder of how technology and nature can work together for our well-being.

Systemic therapies : corticosteroids, immunosuppressants

Systemic therapies are a branch of medical treatment that act on the whole body, often administered orally or by injection. In the field of dermatology, certain serious or recalcitrant skin conditions require more than just topical treatment. This is where corticosteroids and immunosuppressants come into play, offering a more global and often more powerful approach.

Corticosteroids, such as prednisone, are powerful anti-inflammatory agents which reduce the inflammation and symptoms associated with many dermatological conditions. Their action mimics that of the natural hormones produced by the adrenal glands, enabling flare-ups of inflammatory diseases to be rapidly controlled. However, their use is not without side effects, particularly when prolonged. They can affect the body's water and electrolyte balance, impact bone density and trigger mood swings. This is why they are often prescribed for short periods, or in decreasing doses to minimise the risks.

Immunosuppressants such as cyclosporine or methotrexate work by reducing the activity of the immune system. This approach is useful in cases where the immune system mistakenly attacks the skin, as in psoriasis or lupus erythematosus. Although these drugs can offer significant relief, they are not without consequences. Suppressing immunity can make the body more vulnerable to infection. In addition, some of these drugs can affect kidney or liver function.

Nurses, who are on the front line of patient care, play a crucial role in the education and monitoring of patients treated with these systemic therapies. They ensure that patients fully understand the treatment, its benefits and its risks. They are also the sentinels who monitor side effects, guiding patients on their therapeutic journey.

Systemic therapies offer a potentially life-saving solution for many patients suffering from serious skin conditions. However, as there is a flip side to every coin, their use requires careful monitoring and close collaboration between the patient and the medical team to ensure the best balance between efficacy and safety.

Biological therapies and new advances

The advent of biological therapies has truly revolutionised the landscape of dermatological treatment, opening the door to targeted and often more effective interventions for diseases previously considered incurable or difficult to manage. Rather than adopting an 'all-encompassing' approach as with traditional therapies, biological treatments focus on the specific mechanisms at the root of skin diseases.

Biological therapies, often administered in the form of injections, are proteins that target certain parts of the immune system. In the context of diseases such as psoriasis or atopic dermatitis, they act by neutralising the specific inflammatory components that trigger and maintain the disease. For example, some biologics target TNF-alpha, a pro-inflammatory molecule, while others attack specific interleukins.

What makes these therapies so promising is their ability to offer rapid and lasting relief, often with fewer side effects than traditional systemic treatments. However, because they modify the activity of the immune system, they can also increase the risk of infections.

In addition to biological therapies, dermatology is experiencing other exciting advances. Gene therapy, for example, which involves introducing or modifying genes in a patient's cells to treat or prevent a disease, is currently being explored for certain hereditary skin conditions. Artificial intelligence and telemedicine are also gaining ground, offering more accurate diagnostic tools and greater access to dermatological care.

Nurses, always on the frontier between patient and medicine, play a central role in this new era. They are trained in the latest advances, ensuring that patients benefit from the most effective treatments while guaranteeing their safety. What's more, their role as educators is growing, as they help patients navigate this constantly changing medical landscape.

The world of dermatology is in full swing, with advances transforming the way we understand and treat skin diseases. As part of this dynamic, nurses are positioning themselves as beacons of light, guiding patients towards ever more promising therapeutic horizons.

Chapter 7:
MANAGING DERMATOLOGICAL EMERGENCIES

Burns and traumatic injuries

Burns and traumatic skin injuries are among the most common and delicate conditions to treat in dermatology. They cover a wide range of injuries, from minor scrapes to deep burns, each type requiring specific management to ensure optimal healing.

Burns can be classified according to their severity: from first degree, which only affects the outer layer of the skin, to fourth degree, which can damage muscles, tendons and sometimes even bones. The source of the burn is also varied: thermal (hot or cold), chemical, electrical or radiation.

The management of burns is a delicate matter. It requires a rapid assessment of the depth and extent of the injury to decide on the best therapeutic approach. Superficial burns can often be treated with soothing ointments and dressings, while deeper burns may require hospitalisation, skin grafts or even reconstructive surgery.

Traumatic injuries, on the other hand, are generally caused by physical accidents, such as cuts, abrasions or grazes. Like burns, they require careful assessment to determine the best treatment approach. This can range from simple dressings and sutures to more specialised wound care to prevent infection and minimise scarring.

The dermatology nurse plays an essential role in the management of these lesions. They are often the first point of contact for the patient, assessing the severity of the lesion, providing first aid and referring the patient to specialist care if necessary. In addition, they follow up patients, monitoring healing, changing dressings, identifying signs of infection and offering advice on home care.

But beyond these technical skills, nurses also provide emotional support. Burns and traumatic injuries can be painful, frightening and sometimes disfiguring. Nurses reassure patients, listen to them and support them on their road to recovery, looking after not only their physical health, but also their psychological well-being.

Burns and traumatic lesions require care that is both scientific and humane. In this delicate ballet of care, the dermatology nurse is a central figure, combining skill, compassion and dedication to guide the patient towards complete recovery.

Acute allergic reactions

Acute allergic skin reactions, known as urticaria or angioedema depending on their location and intensity, are sudden and often unexpected skin manifestations resulting from the body's hypersensitivity to an allergenic agent. Whether it's an insect sting, a medicine, a food, or even an environmental trigger such as pollen, skin responses can be both alarming and potentially dangerous.

Hives manifest themselves as red, raised, itchy patches that can appear anywhere on the body. These lesions can vary in size, from small patches to large plaques, and can move or coalesce over time. Sometimes the reaction is accompanied by deeper swelling, often in the lips, eyelids or throat, known as angioedema.

Immediate treatment is essential. If the reaction is mild, antihistamines can be given to calm the itching and reduce inflammation. However, if the reaction is severe or affects breathing, emergency medical intervention is required, including the administration of epinephrine to counteract the reaction.

The dermatology nurse is often the first healthcare professional to assess and treat these reactions. They must be able to quickly distinguish between a benign reaction and one that could be life-threatening. Once the acute crisis has been managed, the nurse plays a crucial role in educating the patient, helping them to identify and avoid trigger allergens, understand the need to carry an emergency kit in the case of severe allergies, and recognise the early signs of an allergic reaction so they can act quickly.

But beyond medical treatment, nurses also provide emotional support. An acute allergic reaction can be traumatic, leaving the patient with a persistent fear of future triggers. The nurse reassures, answers questions and provides practical advice to help the patient manage and prevent possible future reactions.
When faced with acute allergic reactions, the dermatology nurse skilfully combines clinical skills, proactive education and empathy, guaranteeing comprehensive care that goes beyond the simple cutaneous response, and delves deeply into the patient's overall well-being.

Conditions requiring rapid intervention

In dermatology, certain conditions require rapid treatment because of their potential seriousness or rapid evolution. These emergency situations may be the result of infections, inflammatory conditions, cancers or other underlying pathologies. For the dermatology nurse, being able to recognise and intervene in these situations is crucial.

1. Erysipelas and infectious cellulitis:
Erysipelas is an acute bacterial skin infection caused mainly by streptococcus. It manifests itself as intense redness, swelling, heat and pain. Infectious cellulitis is similar, but affects the deeper layers of the skin. Without prompt treatment, the infection can spread rapidly and become potentially fatal.

2. Necrotizing fasciitis:
This is a rare but fearsome infection that rapidly destroys the soft tissue under the skin. The initial symptoms can be deceptive, but the pain is often disproportionate to the initial appearance of the skin.

3. Pemphigus vulgaris:
This is an autoimmune disease that causes blisters to form on the skin and mucous membranes. If left untreated, this condition can cause serious complications.

4. Melanoma:
This is a type of skin cancer which, when detected at an early stage, is highly treatable. However, if allowed to progress, melanoma can rapidly metastasise to other parts of the body.

5. Serious drug reactions:
Some skin reactions to medicines can be severe and potentially fatal, such as Stevens-Johnson syndrome or toxic epidermal necrolysis. These conditions manifest themselves as desquamation and a painful skin rash, and require hospitalisation.

For the dermatology nurse, early recognition of these pathologies is crucial. Intervention must be rapid to minimise damage and maximise the chances of recovery.

In addition to diagnosis and treatment, patient education on the signs and symptoms to watch out for is fundamental, especially in conditions where the risk of recurrence is high.

The nurse is often the emotional pillar for the patient in an emergency situation. The ability to reassure, listen and inform is just as essential as clinical skills. In short, within the spectrum of dermatological pathologies, these emergencies are a reminder of the crucial importance of rapid intervention and clinical excellence in care.

Chapter 8:
PAEDIATRIC DERMATOLOGY

Special features of children's skin

Children's skin is unique, and this uniqueness extends far beyond its softness to the touch. From a dermatological perspective, understanding these specific characteristics is essential if we are to offer optimum care to this young population.

1. Thickness:
The skin of newborns and young children is thinner than that of adults. This makes their skin more vulnerable to infection, irritation and the effects of the sun. It is also less resistant to rubbing or trauma.

2. Water content:
Children's skin has a different hydration capacity. Although it can retain water effectively, it also loses it more quickly, making children more susceptible to skin dehydration.

3. Melanin production:
Melanin production in children, particularly newborns, is not as efficient as in adults, making them more sensitive to UV rays.

4. Barrier function:
Because it is so thin, children's skin barrier is less effective, which can lead to increased absorption of external substances. This makes them more sensitive to topical products, allergens and other environmental agents.

5. Production of sweat:

Children's sweat glands are not fully functional from birth. This can affect their ability to regulate body temperature effectively by sweating.

6. Sensitivity:
Children's skin is more sensitive to irritation and inflammation. Conditions such as eczema, nappy dermatitis and other skin rashes are more common in young children.

7. Healing:
Although children's skin has a great capacity for regeneration, the healing process can be different. The formation of hypertrophic or keloid scars may be more frequent in some children.

As healthcare professionals, understanding these nuances is vital when it comes to the dermatological care of children. Treatment choices, frequency of care, prevention and parent education all need to be adapted to these particularities. Every stage, from assessment to prescription and education, requires a child-centred approach, ensuring safe, effective care that is tailored to their specific needs.

Common ailments in children

In children, a number of dermatological conditions are particularly prevalent or specific to this age group. These skin disorders are often the result of a combination of factors, including the peculiarities of the child's skin, his or her developing immune system, environment and interactions. The following is a non-exhaustive list of skin disorders commonly seen in children:

1. Eczema or atopic dermatitis:
This is a chronic skin condition characterised by red patches, itching and dry skin. It can appear as early as the first few months of life and is often linked to other atopic symptoms such as asthma or hay fever.

2. Chickenpox:
This viral disease is typical of childhood and manifests itself as a skin rash of itchy vesicles that develop into scabs.

3. Seborrhoeic dermatitis (cradle cap):
This is a common condition in infants, manifesting itself as scaly, oily patches on the scalp, but can also affect the face and other areas of the body.

4. Molloscum contagiosum:
These are small skin papules, generally benign, caused by a virus. They can appear anywhere on the body, but are often concentrated in areas of friction.

5. Impetigo:
This is a superficial bacterial infection, often caused by staphylococcus aureus or streptococcus, characterised by oozing lesions and honey-coloured crusts.

6. Warts:
These benign skin growths are caused by the human papillomavirus (HPV) and can appear on the hands, feet or other parts of the body.

7. Urticaria:
Raised red patches, often itchy, which may be caused by food allergies, infections or other triggers.

8. Roseola:
It is a viral disease characterised by a high fever followed by a pale pink rash.

9. Diaper rash:
This skin irritation is common in babies and toddlers, generally as a reaction to dampness or rubbing of nappies.

10. Café-au-lait stains:
These are benign pigment spots, light brown in colour, which often appear from birth or during the first few years of life.

Understanding these conditions and their typical presentations is crucial for the dermatology nurse working with children. Management often involves a combination of medical treatment and parent education on home care, prevention and follow-up. Each condition, although common, requires detailed attention to ensure the child's well-being and to reassure parents.

Communication and specific care for young patients

Dermatological management of young patients is not just about medical treatment or direct care. Communication and an age-specific approach are crucial to a positive medical experience for both the child and his or her parents or guardians.

1. Child-centred approach :
When caring for a young patient, it is essential to involve them as much as possible in the care process. Children should be treated with respect, taking into account their level of understanding and ability to participate in decisions about their care.

2. Creating a reassuring environment :
Medical facilities can be intimidating for children. So it's important to create a welcoming environment, with age-appropriate toys, books and visual distractions.

3. Age-appropriate communication :
It is essential to use clear, simple language that is appropriate to the child's age. Explaining the procedures to come, using simple analogies or toys to show what is going to happen can help to alleviate fears.

4. Involvement of parents or guardians :
Parents play an essential role in the care process. Make sure they understand diagnosis, treatment and home care. Encourage them to ask questions and to be active partners in their child's care.

5. Distraction techniques :
Using distraction techniques during procedures or treatments can reduce anxiety and pain. This can include the use of music, videos, books or even breathing techniques.

6. Respect the child's rhythm :
Every child is unique. Some may need more time to adapt to the medical environment or to become comfortable with a procedure. Respecting their rhythm and giving them the time they need is crucial.

7. Further training :
It is essential for dermatology nurses to receive ongoing training on best practice in paediatric communication and the management of young patients.

8. Feedback and adjustments :
Ask for regular feedback from the children and their parents. This information can help identify areas for

improvement and adapt the approach or communication techniques.

9. Emotional support :
Acknowledge and validate the child's feelings. Some may be worried, frightened or frustrated by their condition or medical procedures. Emotional support is just as important as physical care.

The key to success in the dermatological management of young patients lies in a combination of clinical skills, appropriate communication and genuine empathy for each child's unique experience. Together, these elements can create a positive medical experience and promote optimal outcomes.

Chapter 9: COSMETIC DERMATOLOGY AND SURGICAL

Common cosmetic procedures

Cosmetic procedures in dermatology have seen a significant increase in popularity in recent years, largely due to technological advances that make them safer and more effective. These procedures are often designed to improve the appearance of the skin, reduce the signs of ageing and enhance aesthetic features. Here is an overview of common cosmetic procedures in dermatology:

1. Botulinum toxin (Botox) :
Injected into the facial muscles, it is used to reduce the appearance of dynamic wrinkles such as forehead wrinkles or crow's feet near the eyes.

2. Dermal fillers :
These gels, often hyaluronic acid-based, are injected to fill in wrinkles, redefine facial contours and restore volume, particularly on the cheeks, lips and nasolabial fold.

3. Chemical peel :
This involves using a chemical solution to exfoliate the surface layer of the skin, reducing the appearance of pigment spots, fine lines and other imperfections.

4. Microdermabrasion :
An exfoliation technique that uses tiny crystals to remove the top layer of dead skin, leaving skin softer and brighter.

5. Laser therapy :
There are different types of lasers used to treat pigment spots, scars, wrinkles, visible blood vessels and even skin resurfacing.

6. Intense pulsed light (IPL) :
Used to treat pigmentation spots, rosacea, visible blood vessels and other skin imperfections.

7. Laser hair removal :
A laser beam targets the hair follicles to reduce the growth of unwanted hair.

8. Cryolipolysis :
A non-invasive method that uses cold to break down fat cells without damaging the surrounding tissue.

9. Sclerotherapy :
A treatment for spider veins in which a solution is injected into the veins, causing them to shrink.

10. Radiofrequency therapy :
It uses radio waves to heat the dermis, stimulating collagen production and tightening the skin.

11. Microneedling :
Small needles create micro-injuries in the skin, stimulating the production of collagen and elastin.

12. Hair transplants :
For those suffering from baldness or thinning hair, individual follicular units can be transplanted from one part of the scalp to another.

13. Combination therapies :
Dermatologists often combine different procedures to obtain optimum results, such as a chemical peel followed by laser therapy.

These procedures, although aesthetically pleasing, require precise expertise and careful patient assessment. A thorough initial consultation, where expectations and risks are clearly discussed, is crucial to ensure patient safety and satisfaction.

Surgical techniques in dermatology

Dermatological surgery covers a wide range of procedures, from minor interventions to more complex surgeries. These techniques are mainly used to treat skin lesions, whether benign, precancerous or malignant. Here is an overview of the surgical techniques commonly used in dermatology:

1. Surgical excision :
This is the removal of a skin lesion using a scalpel. After excision, the edges of the wound are sutured. This technique is frequently used to remove cysts, lipomas and certain skin tumours.

2. Mohs surgery :
This is a precise surgical technique used to treat skin cancers, in particular basal cell carcinoma and squamous cell carcinoma. It involves removing the tumour layer by layer, checking each layer under a microscope until no more cancerous cells are detected.

3. Curettage and electrocautery :
After scraping a lesion with a curette, an electrode is used to cauterise the area and stop the bleeding. This is often used to treat seborrhoeic keratoses and certain superficial carcinomas.

4. Skin biopsy :
A small portion of tissue is removed for examination under a microscope. There are various biopsy techniques, such as punch biopsy, shave biopsy or excisional biopsy.

5. Cryosurgery :
Using liquid nitrogen, this technique 'freezes' and destroys skin lesions. It is commonly used for warts, actinic keratoses and other benign lesions.

6. Surgical lasers :
Some lasers are used to remove skin lesions, treat varicose veins or resurface the skin.

7. Skin grafting :
When a large area of skin is lost or damaged, a skin graft may be necessary. Skin can be taken from another part of the patient's body.

8. Skin flap :
Unlike grafts, skin flaps have their own blood supply. They are used to cover loss of substance, particularly after Mohs surgery.

9. Liposuction :
Although most commonly associated with cosmetic surgery, liposuction can also be used in dermatology to treat conditions such as lipoedema.

10. Dermabrasion :
This is a mechanical resurfacing of the skin to treat acne scars, wrinkles and other imperfections.

11. Drainage and incision of abscesses :
In the event of a skin infection forming an abscess, an incision may be made to drain the pus.

Dermatological surgery requires great precision, specific expertise and a thorough assessment of the lesions. The prevention of complications, post-operative follow-up and effective communication with the patient are essential to the success of these operations.

Post-operative care and preventing complications

Post-operative care is crucial to ensure optimal healing after dermatological surgery. Good care not only ensures that the wound heals, but also minimises scarring and prevents complications.

Here is a fluid presentation on the subject:
After dermatological surgery, post-operative care plays a fundamental role for the patient. An incision, even a minor one, represents an open door to the body, and it is imperative to ensure that healing takes place under the best possible conditions.
Cleaning the wound: Cleanliness is the first line of defence against infection. It is essential to gently clean the operated area with a mild antiseptic solution, as recommended by the dermatologist. Avoid aggressive rubbing that could damage the fragile area.
Dressings: Depending on the nature and location of the operation, sterile dressings will be required. They play a protective role, preventing contamination of the wound and absorbing any exudation. These dressings must be changed regularly and whenever they become wet or soiled.
Antibiotics: In some cases, to prevent infection, a course of topical or oral antibiotics may be prescribed. It is crucial to follow the recommended dosage and not to interrupt treatment prematurely.

Pain management: If pain occurs after the operation, painkillers may be prescribed. However, it is important to avoid drugs that can promote bleeding, such as aspirin.

Reducing swelling: After certain operations, swelling can occur. Using cold compresses or elevating the operated area can help reduce inflammation.

Limiting physical activity: To avoid stress on the wound and promote optimal healing, it may be necessary to limit certain movements or activities for a set period of time.

Sun protection: Newly-operated skin is particularly sensitive to UV rays. Sun protection is therefore essential to prevent hyperpigmentation or discolouration of the scar.

Monitoring: Any abnormal signs, such as excessive redness, oozing, local heat or increased pain, should be reported promptly. These are potential indicators of complications, such as infection.

Moisturising and caring for the scar: Once the wound has healed properly, regular application of a moisturising cream or specific product can improve the appearance of the scar.

Preventing complications depends largely on close collaboration between the patient and the healthcare professional. By scrupulously respecting post-operative advice and maintaining open communication with their dermatologist, patients maximise their chances of a smooth recovery and a satisfactory aesthetic result.

Chapter 10:
CHALLENGES AND ETHICS IN DERMATOLOGY

Patient management with chronic illnesses

Managing patients with chronic skin diseases requires a holistic approach, taking into account not only the physical aspects of the disease, but also the psychological, social and emotional implications it can have. Here is a fluid exploration of the management of these patients:

As the body's largest organ and a visible interface with the outside world, the skin plays an essential role in our identity and self-perception. When it is affected by a chronic disease, this can have a profound impact on the patient's quality of life.

Comprehensive assessment: The first step in treatment is a comprehensive assessment of the nature, severity and impact of the skin condition. This assessment includes a detailed medical history, clinical examination and, if necessary, diagnostic tests.

Individualised treatment plan: Every patient is unique, and it is essential to develop a treatment plan tailored to their specific needs. This may include topical medications, systemic therapies, phototherapy sessions or even surgery.

Psychological support: Chronic skin diseases can have a considerable impact on a patient's emotional well-being. Offering psychological support, whether through individual consultations or support groups, is essential. In some cases, follow-up with a psychologist or psychiatrist may be beneficial.

Patient education : Self-management is a key component of chronic disease management. Educating patients about their disease, available treatments and self-care measures can significantly improve adherence to treatment and quality of life.

Regular monitoring: Chronic diseases require ongoing monitoring to assess the effectiveness of treatment, identify any complications and adjust the care plan accordingly.

Open communication: A relationship of trust between the patient and the care team is essential. Open communication ensures that the patient's concerns, questions and needs are addressed and taken into account.

Managing exacerbations: Chronic illnesses can experience periods of exacerbation. Being prepared and knowing how to manage these periods can reduce the associated anxiety and improve outcomes.

Integration of care: Patients with chronic skin diseases may require care from several specialists. Ensuring effective communication and coordination between different care providers is crucial.

Prevention and awareness: Informing patients about potential triggers and preventive measures can help reduce the frequency and severity of flare-ups.

Social implications: Skin diseases can have an impact on a patient's social and professional life. Offering advice on how to manage these challenges is fundamental.

Managing patients with chronic skin diseases requires an empathetic, integrative and evidence-based approach. By focusing on understanding, support and collaboration, healthcare professionals can help these patients lead as normal and fulfilling a life as possible.

Ethical issues related to cosmetology

Cosmetology, which encompasses the study and application of aesthetic treatments to enhance or alter appearance, is a constantly evolving field and subject to a unique set of ethical issues. Here is a fluid exploration of some of the ethical concerns commonly encountered in this field:

The quest for beauty and perfection is almost as old as humanity itself. However, in the age of advanced technology, social media and ubiquitous advertising, this quest has taken on a new dimension. Cosmetology, at the crossroads of medical science, art and commerce, faces a myriad of ethical dilemmas.

Beauty standards: Cosmetology is often influenced by fluctuating beauty standards, conveyed by the media and popular culture. Can these standards lead to undue social pressure or create unrealistic ideals of beauty? And what about promoting diversity and self-acceptance?

Informed consent: Any cosmetic treatment, whether invasive or not, involves risks. Do patients receive all the information they need to make an informed decision? Is a patient's desire for a procedure truly autonomous or is it influenced by external factors?

Access to treatments: Cosmetology is often expensive, which raises the question of equity. Should high-quality aesthetic treatments be accessible to everyone, regardless of their financial ability?

Training and competence: With the growing popularity of aesthetic procedures, many providers are offering services without the necessary training or expertise. How can we guarantee patient safety and professionalism in this field?

Commercial exploitation: The marketing of cosmetology services can sometimes exaggerate the benefits or minimise the risks, leading to unwise decisions. Where do we draw the line between ethical advertising and manipulation?

Research and innovation: Should cosmetology research be subject to the same strict ethical standards as medical research? And how can we ensure that new techniques or products are safe before they are widely adopted?

Psychological repercussions: It is crucial to recognise that not all problems of self-esteem or body perception can be resolved by cosmetic procedures. How can we ensure that patients receive appropriate psychological support before opting for procedures?

Procedures on minors: Cosmetic procedures on minors raise additional ethical questions. To what extent can an adolescent give informed consent for a procedure that will have long-term repercussions?

Sustainable and ethical: In an age of environmental awareness, it is also essential to consider the ecological impact of cosmetic products and procedures. Are they sustainable? Are products tested on animals?

Faced with these dilemmas, cosmetology must constantly evaluate and re-evaluate its practices. Respect for patient autonomy, a commitment to professional integrity and recognition of the wider societal impact of the field are essential to navigating these ethically complex waters.

Continuity of care and psychological support

Continuity of care and psychological support in dermatology, as in other medical disciplines, play a crucial role in ensuring comprehensive, holistic patient care. Let's look at these concepts from a fluid, integrated perspective.

The skin, a silent witness to our lives, is much more than just a shield against the elements. It reflects our history, our health and, in many cases, our inner concerns. Dermatology, therefore, cannot be limited to treating skin disorders: it must also take into account the human being behind the skin.

Continuity of care
Continuity of care refers to coordinated, uninterrupted care that extends well beyond the first consultation. It is essential for :
- **Building trust:** A patient who knows that he or she is regularly monitored by a medical team will be more inclined to adhere to a treatment plan and share his or her concerns.
- **Treating chronic conditions:** Many dermatological conditions, such as psoriasis or eczema, require long-term monitoring. Continuity of care guarantees optimal management adapted to the progression of the disease.
- **Preventing complications:** Regular consultations enable early detection of signs of worsening or the side-effects of treatment, allowing rapid intervention.

Psychological support
The role of psychological support in dermatology is twofold:
- **Managing the emotional impact:** Skin conditions, which are visible and sometimes stigmatising, can have a profound effect on self-esteem, body image and quality of life. Psychological support helps patients to manage these challenges, providing them with the tools to build resilience and well-being.
- **Understanding the underlying cause:** Some skin conditions can be exacerbated by stress or other emotional factors. Psychological support can help identify these triggers and put strategies in place to manage them.

Collaboration between the dermatologist, dermatology nurse and mental health professionals is therefore essential. It makes it possible to offer patients integrated care that goes beyond the simple treatment of skin symptoms to embrace the whole person.

In a world where medicine sometimes tends to be fragmented, continuity of care and psychological support remind us of the importance of seeing the patient as an inseparable whole of body and mind. In dermatology, this holistic approach is not only beneficial, but essential to ensuring patients' long-term well-being.

Chapter 11:
PSYCHOLOGY AND EMOTIONAL SUPPORT

Psychological impact skin disorders

Skin conditions, as visible and often permanent manifestations, can have profound implications for an individual's psychological well-being. Unlike other conditions that may remain invisible to the world, skin problems are often immediately visible, creating a unique set of psychological challenges. Let's delve into the psychological impact of skin conditions.

The skin is much more than just a physical barrier; it is also the mirror of our emotions, our history and, in many ways, our identity. When it is marked by an ailment, this can alter not only our appearance, but also our perception of ourselves.

Stigma and social isolation
Skin conditions can carry a stigma. Conditions such as psoriasis, vitiligo or severe acne can often attract curious looks and even derogatory comments. Some patients may feel judged or misunderstood, which can lead them to isolate themselves socially to avoid judgement.

Self-esteem and body image
The skin plays a crucial role in our body image. Skin conditions can lead to a reduction in self-esteem, particularly in a society where aesthetic perfection is often put on a pedestal. Individuals may feel less attractive, which can affect their confidence in interpersonal and romantic relationships.

Stress and depression
There is a two-way relationship between stress and skin

conditions. Stress can exacerbate many dermatological conditions, while the presence of these conditions can, in turn, increase stress and anxiety levels. In some cases, psychological distress can develop into clinical depression.

Professional repercussions

Some individuals may feel that their skin condition puts them at a disadvantage in the professional world, particularly in professions where appearance plays a central role. This can limit their career opportunities or their desire to progress.

Avoidance behaviour

Shame or embarrassment can lead people with skin conditions to adopt avoidance behaviours: refusing social invitations, avoiding certain activities (such as swimming) or dressing in such a way as to conceal their skin completely.

Recognising the psychological impact of skin conditions is essential if patients are to be offered comprehensive care. Treatment should not only focus on physical symptoms, but also on emotional support, to help patients regain a positive self-image and better manage the impact of their condition on their daily lives.

Holistic approach to the patient : beyond the skin

The holistic approach to the patient in dermatology recognises that each individual is a complex entity, where body, mind and environment constantly interact. While dermatology has traditionally focused on the treatment of skin conditions, a holistic vision goes far beyond the skin, encompassing the emotional, psychological, social and even spiritual impacts of skin diseases on the individual. Let's immerse ourselves in this integrated approach.

Human beings are much more than the sum of their parts; they are multidimensional beings. In dermatology, the holistic approach comes as a reminder that behind every skin condition is a person with his or her own stories, challenges, hopes and fears.

Emotional and psychological dimension
As we explored earlier, skin conditions can have a profound impact on self-esteem, body image and emotional well-being. A holistic approach recognises these challenges and seeks to address them, perhaps by incorporating cognitive-behavioural therapy, relaxation techniques or sessions with a psychologist.

The social dimension
The skin, often regarded as our 'calling card', plays a role in our social interactions. Skin conditions can affect the way an individual interacts with others, isolates themselves or feels stigmatised. Taking a holistic view also means supporting patients in rebuilding their relationships and helping them to navigate the social world with confidence.

The physical dimension
Beyond the apparent skin symptoms, it is essential to understand the underlying causes, which can sometimes be linked to other medical conditions, hormonal imbalances or environmental factors. Healthy eating, exercise and appropriate skin care are also part of this dimension.

Spiritual dimension
For some, their skin and its condition may be linked to deeper questions of meaning, purpose or spirituality. Respecting and exploring this dimension can offer additional support to some patients, helping them to find meaning or acceptance in their condition.

The environmental dimension
The environment plays an essential role in skin health. A holistic approach considers factors such as sun exposure, environmental allergens, air quality and even the cosmetic products used.

A holistic approach to dermatology recognises the patient as a whole. It seeks to treat not only the skin condition, but also to understand and respond to the many challenges patients face in their daily lives. This integrated, patient-centred approach is essential to providing truly transformative and comprehensive care.

Providing emotional support and tailored advice

Emotional support and appropriate advice are key elements of patient care, particularly in the field of dermatology. The appearance of the skin, as a major element of a person's visual identity, can have a profound effect on psychological well-being. Here's how emotional support and appropriate advice can be integrated into patient care with compassion and professionalism.

Empathetic listening
One of the first steps in providing emotional support is to simply listen to the patient. By giving the patient the space and time to share their concerns, fears and frustrations, the nurse or doctor establishes a relationship of trust.

Validating feelings
The emotions associated with skin conditions can be complex. It is essential to validate the patient's feelings, recognise that their concerns are legitimate and never minimise their experiences.

Providing information
Uncertainty and lack of information can exacerbate anxiety. Providing clear, understandable and honest information about the diagnosis, treatment and expectations can help reduce patient anxiety.

Stress management techniques
Learning simple stress management techniques, such as

deep breathing, meditation or journaling, can provide additional emotional support.
Support groups and therapy
Referring patients to support groups specific to their skin condition or to mental health professionals can provide them with valuable resources for managing their emotions.
Advice on personal care
In addition to medical treatments, providing advice on skin care, suitable routines and recommended products can help patients feel more in control of their condition.
Managing expectations
It is essential to discuss the expected results of treatment honestly. If a patient has unrealistic expectations, it is crucial to realign them to avoid future disappointment.
Ongoing training
Ongoing training for healthcare professionals in the psychological aspects of skin disorders can improve the quality of care provided.

The management of skin conditions goes far beyond physical treatment. Recognising and responding to patients' emotional needs is just as crucial to ensuring a comprehensive and empathetic approach to care. By integrating emotional support and tailored advice into the care pathway, professionals can help patients navigate their challenges with confidence and hope.

Chapter 12:
DIVERSITY AND SPECIFIC SKIN CARE

Ethnic differences and specificities skin care

The skin, our body's largest organ, is unique to each of us and bears traces of our origins, heredity and history. Skin characteristics, including colour, texture and reactivity, vary between ethnic groups, which can influence skin conditions, their diagnosis and treatment. This is why understanding ethnic differences and the specificities of skin care is essential to providing appropriate and effective dermatological care.

Skin characteristics by ethnic group

Pigmentation: People of African, Asian or Latin American descent generally have skin richer in melanin, which gives them natural protection against the sun's UV rays. However, this also makes them more susceptible to pigmentation disorders such as post-inflammatory hyperpigmentation.

Texture and pores: Differences in texture and pore size can influence the prevalence of certain skin conditions. For example, Asian skin is often considered to have finer pores, which can influence the way it reacts to certain beauty treatments.

Sensitivity: Certain ethnic groups may be more sensitive to certain skin conditions or react differently to treatments.

Skin conditions and treatments by ethnic group

Pigmentation disorders: Treatments to lighten hyperpigmented areas should be used with caution to avoid causing depigmentation or uneven pigmentation.

- **Scarring**: People with darker skin are sometimes more prone to keloid or hypertrophic scarring. Treatments must be adapted to minimise this risk.
- **Ageing**: The way in which the skin ages can vary according to ethnic group, with differences in the appearance of wrinkles, skin laxity and brown spots.

Specific features of skin care

- **Sun protection**: Even though darker skins have a natural protection against UV rays, the use of a sunscreen remains essential to prevent skin cancer and pigmentation disorders.
- **Lightening products**: It is crucial to choose products formulated to minimise irritation and prevent pigmentation disorders.
- **Moisturising care**: Black skin can often look "ashy" when dry. Regular use of suitable moisturisers is beneficial.

Providing appropriate dermatological care requires a thorough understanding of ethnic differences and the specificities of skin care. Healthcare professionals need to continually educate themselves and listen to their patients to meet their unique needs and ensure the best possible results.

Pigmentation disorders and specific concerns

Pigmentation disorders encompass a wide range of skin conditions characterised by abnormal skin pigmentation. These disorders can be the result of increased, decreased or poorly distributed production of melanin, the pigment responsible for colouring the skin, hair and eyes. These conditions can have a significant impact on an individual's self-esteem and quality of life, due to their visibility and sometimes permanent nature.

The main pigmentation disorders

Melasma: Also known as "pregnancy mask", this is a brown or greyish hyperpigmentation that generally appears on the face. It is common in pregnant women, users of oral contraceptives and those taking hormone replacement therapy.

Post-inflammatory hyperpigmentation (PIH): This is a skin reaction to inflammation or injury, which can follow conditions such as acne, rashes or wounds. It can appear as dark patches on the skin.

Vitiligo: This is a disorder in which portions of the skin lose their pigmentation, forming discoloured areas. The exact causes remain a subject of research, but a genetic predisposition and an auto-immune reaction appear to be involved.

Freckles and lentigines: These small brown spots are generally caused by sun exposure and are more common in fair-skinned individuals.

Albinism: This is a genetic condition resulting in a total or partial absence of melanin in the skin, hair and eyes.

Specific concerns related to pigmentation disorders

Psychological impact: Individuals may experience feelings of embarrassment, shame or lack of self-confidence due to the visibility of pigmentation disorders.

Sensitivity to the sun: Areas affected by conditions such as vitiligo are more sensitive to the sun, increasing the risk of sunburn and skin cancer.

Choice of treatment: The choice of treatment for pigmentation disorders must be individualised and carried out with caution, as certain treatments, if not properly managed, can aggravate hyperpigmentation or cause other adverse effects.

Prevention: In some cases, active prevention is possible. For example, avoiding excessive exposure to the sun can prevent melasma from worsening.

Pigmentation disorders, although often not life-threatening, can have a profound impact on an individual's well-being. Holistic care, including clinical assessment, tailored treatments, psychological support and advice on prevention and daily care, is essential to help patients manage these conditions and regain their self-confidence.

Tackling diversity with sensitivity and skill

Embracing diversity with sensitivity and skill is not only a necessity in our modern interconnected world, but also a virtue. In a society where our neighbours, colleagues and friends come from diverse backgrounds, understanding and respecting differences is fundamental to building a harmonious community. Each individual brings with them a mosaic of experiences, traditions and perspectives that enrich the collective tapestry of our humanity.

The essence of sensitivity to diversity lies in the recognition that each person is unique and has their own story to tell. It's not just about skin colour, ethnic origin or religious belief. It's also about gender, sexual orientation, age, physical and mental abilities, education and so many other facets that shape our identity. By adopting an open approach, asking questions with curiosity and listening attentively, we begin to understand the experiences of others, dismantle stereotypes and eliminate prejudice.

Competence, on the other hand, requires continuous education. In a constantly changing world, it is essential to be proactive in seeking out information, attending training courses and taking part in dialogues on diversity. This enables us not only to become familiar with different cultures and traditions, but also to understand the challenges faced by certain communities. This skill helps us to interact more respectfully and effectively with people from different backgrounds.

But dealing with diversity sensitively and competently goes beyond simple personal interaction. It also extends to our workplaces, our schools and our communities. By creating inclusive environments, promoting diversity and offering equal opportunities to all, we are building solid structures that reflect the rich diversity of our society. Ultimately, sensitivity to diversity and competence are not just individual qualities, but also the pillars on which a balanced, fair and thriving society is built.

Chapter 13:
TECHNOLOGY IN DERMATOLOGY

The latest diagnostic tools

Dermatology, like many branches of medicine, has undergone a remarkable evolution in terms of diagnostic tools over the last few decades. Technological advances have made it possible to improve diagnostic accuracy, offer non-invasive solutions and optimise patient management. In a fluid style, let's explore some of the most recent diagnostic tools in dermatology.

The **dermatoscope** has become a must-have for many dermatologists. It is an optical device that enables the skin to be examined on an enlarged scale. Thanks to dermatoscopy, doctors can identify skin structures that are invisible to the naked eye, improving the early detection of melanoma and other skin tumours.

Another technological leap has been the implementation of **optical coherence tomography (OCT) imaging**. This technique offers cross-sectional images of the skin, providing details similar to a microscopic biopsy, but without the need for surgery. OCT is particularly useful for monitoring disease progression and the effectiveness of treatments.

Multispectral imaging is an innovative method that uses different wavelengths of light to examine the skin. It is capable of detecting changes in tissue long before they become visible to the naked eye, thus helping in the early detection of various skin conditions.

Raman spectroscopy is an emerging technique that analyses molecular vibrations to obtain information about the biochemical composition of tissues. Although still under development, it could revolutionise the diagnosis of diseases such as skin cancer.

Finally, **artificial intelligence** (AI) and machine learning are beginning to play a role in dermatology. By combining vast databases of skin images with powerful algorithms, AI can help identify diseases with an accuracy sometimes equal to or greater than that of human experts. Although this technology is still in its infancy in dermatology, its potential is undeniable.

Diagnostic tools in dermatology have come a long way, offering healthcare professionals more accurate, rapid and non-invasive ways of examining and treating skin conditions. As technology continues to evolve, we can expect these tools to become even more sophisticated, transforming the way we approach skin health.

Telemedicine and consultation remotely

Telemedicine, the fusion of technology and medicine, has become an essential pillar of the modern medical landscape. In particular, in the context of dermatology, remote consultation has opened up new avenues for the delivery of care. Let's take a fluid approach to this subject, highlighting the growing importance of telemedicine and remote consultation in dermatology.

Imagine a world where, faced with a worrying skin rash or a changing mole, you don't have to wait weeks for an appointment in person. Thanks to telemedicine, that world is our reality today. With a simple photo or a brief video conference, you can have a direct exchange with your dermatologist, benefiting from a rapid and often accurate diagnosis.

Telemedicine not only meets the need for convenience, but also for accessibility. For those who live in remote areas or have difficulty travelling, remote consultations are a lifeline. This method of delivering medical care eliminates geographical barriers, making dermatology accessible to everyone, regardless of where they live.

The effectiveness of telemedicine in dermatology is enhanced by the visual nature of the speciality. A picture is often worth a thousand words, especially when it comes to skin problems. Dermatologists can assess, diagnose and even prescribe treatment based on high-resolution images or videos in real time, reducing the need for face-to-face consultations in many cases.

However, telemedicine also has its challenges. The absence of a direct physical examination can sometimes limit diagnosis. In addition, concerns about patient confidentiality and data security require constant attention to ensure that telemedicine platforms are both secure and compliant.

Despite these challenges, the future of telemedicine in dermatology looks promising. With the continuing evolution of technology, appropriate training for healthcare professionals, and well thought-out regulations, telemedicine is set to revolutionise the way in which dermatological care is delivered.

Telemedicine and remote consultation have transformed dermatology, making it more accessible and convenient for patients around the world. As this modality of care continues to flourish, it is redefining our perception of medical care, demonstrating that sometimes optimal care can be delivered even from miles away.

Electronic file management and care coordination

The advent of the digital age has brought about a radical transformation in the medical field, notably with the implementation of electronic medical record management. At the heart of this evolution is the ambition to offer better, more consistent and more effective care to all patients. In dermatology, as in other medical specialities, this transition to digital technology has had a profound impact, facilitating not only the management of records but also the coordination of care.

Electronic records management has put an end to the piles of paper files, the often illegible handwritten notes and heavy filing cabinets that once characterised doctors' surgeries. Instead, doctors, nurses and other healthcare professionals can now access complete, clearly organised and regularly updated records in just a few clicks. These electronic records, containing images, laboratory reports and medical histories, become invaluable tools for diagnosis, follow-up and treatment.

But beyond simply managing records, these electronic systems play a crucial role in coordinating care. Take, for example, a psoriasis patient who requires both dermatological and rheumatological care. Thanks to an electronically shared medical file, doctors from different specialities can work more closely together, ensuring that the patient receives comprehensive, consistent care. They can discuss treatments, exchange relevant information and ensure that the patient receives optimum care at every stage of his or her treatment.

What's more, these systems encourage direct communication with patients. Patient portals, for example, allow individuals to access their own medical records, book appointments online, and even ask questions of their carers. This patient-centred approach builds trust, improves understanding and encourages greater adherence to treatment.

However, like any innovation, electronic records management also presents challenges. Security and confidentiality issues are at the forefront, requiring rigorous protocols to protect sensitive information. In addition, the need for ongoing training for staff and adaptation to new systems can represent initial obstacles.

Electronic case management and care coordination have redefined modern dermatology practice. Although still a work in progress, this digital revolution promises continuous improvements in the quality of care, greater collaboration between healthcare professionals and an even stronger patient-caregiver relationship. In this constantly changing landscape, the goal remains unchanged: to offer the best possible care to every patient.

Chapter 14:
PREVENTION AND EDUCATION

Raising awareness of the dangers of the sun and sun protection

The sun, that eternal ball of fire shining in the sky, has always been associated with life, warmth and light. We marvel at it, we bask in it, and yet, like all good things, it has a downside. In dermatology, awareness of the dangers of the sun and the importance of sun protection are crucial subjects that deserve sustained attention.

The sun emits a variety of rays, including ultraviolet (UV) rays which, although invisible to the naked eye, have a profound effect on our skin. Repeated, unprotected exposure to UV rays can damage the skin's DNA, accelerate skin ageing and, most importantly, increase the risk of skin cancers such as melanoma. Every year, thousands of new cases of skin cancer are diagnosed, many of them directly linked to overexposure to the sun without adequate protection.

But how, in a society that touts a tanned complexion as a symbol of health and beauty, can we effectively raise awareness of these dangers? First and foremost, it's a question of education. It's essential to teach people about the potential harmful effects of the sun from an early age. Schools, the media and public health campaigns can play a decisive role in raising awareness.

At the same time, sun protection should not be seen as a constraint, but as a daily ritual, in the same way as brushing your teeth or washing your hands. Regular use of broad-spectrum sun creams with a sun protection factor

(SPF) suited to your skin type and sun conditions is essential. It is also advisable to wear protective clothing, wide-brimmed hats and sunglasses, and to avoid direct exposure during the hours when the sun is strongest.

It's also important to dispel certain myths. A tan is not a sign of healthy skin; it's actually the skin's response to being attacked by UV rays. Similarly, tanned skin does not offer sufficient protection against the dangers of the sun. Each sunburn, each intensive tanning session, accumulates and increases the risk of long-term harmful effects.

The sun, although a source of life, also brings with it dangers that should not be overlooked. Increased awareness of the risks associated with unprotected exposure, coupled with rigorous sun protection habits, can save lives. After all, the best way to enjoy the sun is to do so safely, with awareness and respect for this powerful force of nature.

Skin self-examination and early detection

The skin, that vast expanse that envelops our body, is much more than just a protective barrier. It tells our story, reveals our experiences, and sometimes silently signals changes that could have serious implications for our health. Skin self-examination and early detection of skin abnormalities are proving to be powerful tools in the prevention and treatment of skin diseases, including cancer.

Every day, our skin is exposed to a multitude of environmental factors, from sun and wind to pollutants. Over time, these factors can induce changes, sometimes imperceptible, sometimes more marked. And while most of these changes are harmless, some can be the first signs of more serious conditions. Regular self-examination of the skin allows these changes to be spotted early, increasing the chances of successful treatment.

Self-examination is a simple ritual, but it requires rigour and attention. It involves standing in front of a mirror, preferably in natural light, and inspecting every square centimetre of your skin, from head to toe. It's essential to pay attention to the appearance of new spots, changes in the appearance or size of existing moles, or any lesions that don't heal. Every detail counts, because the slightest change can be revealing.

It is also crucial to know your own skin type and history. Fair skin, for example, is generally more susceptible to sun damage, and therefore to skin cancer. Similarly, a family history of skin cancer can increase a person's risk. This information can help focus attention during self-examinations.

But why is it so important to detect these changes early? Because in the world of dermatology, time is of the essence. The earlier an abnormality is detected, the better the chances of treatment and cure. Take melanoma, for example, one of the most aggressive skin cancers. If detected at an early stage, the five-year survival rate is over 90%. However, if the diagnosis is made late, this rate can drop drastically.

Skin self-examination is an act of empowerment, a proactive way of taking control of our own health. It's a reminder that our skin, with all its complexity and beauty, needs our attention and care. By listening to what our skin has to tell us, by spotting even the most discreet signals, we give ourselves the best chance of living a healthy, beautiful and fulfilled life.

Patient education on daily skin care

The skin is the largest organ in the human body, and although it may often appear resilient and self-sufficient, it requires regular care and attention to maintain its health and vitality. Educating patients about daily skin care is not just a question of aesthetics; it is first and foremost a proactive approach to maintaining skin health, preventing skin disorders and optimising its protective function.

When we talk about skin care, the first thing that often comes to mind is a beauty routine, with its lotions and potions. But skincare is much more than creams and serums. It's a holistic approach that encompasses protection, nutrition and skin renewal.

Protecting the skin is essential, especially in the face of external aggression. This includes protection against the sun's UV rays, which can cause irreversible damage to the skin, accelerate skin ageing and increase the risk of skin cancers. Educating patients about the importance of applying a broad-spectrum sun cream every day, even on cloudy days, is crucial. Similarly, it is important to raise awareness of the harmful effects of pollutants, tobacco and other environmental factors, while advising appropriate methods of protection.

Skin nutrition is just as important. Well-hydrated skin is radiant, supple and resistant. Informing patients about the importance of hydration, both by applying appropriate moisturising products and by drinking enough water, is a fundamental step. In addition, promoting a balanced diet rich in antioxidants, vitamins and minerals helps to nourish the skin from within, making it more resilient in the face of everyday challenges.

Finally, the skin, like any living organ, has a life cycle. Encouraging gentle exfoliation routines to eliminate dead cells and promote cell renewal is essential. Educating people about the importance of skin care tailored to different skin types and conditions, from oily skin to sensitive skin, ensures personalised care.

Educating patients about daily skin care means giving them the tools to take charge of their skin's health, to protect, nourish and renew it. It's a journey towards better health, greater self-confidence and, inevitably, a better quality of life.

Chapter 15:
ADMINISTRATIVE AND MANAGEMENT ASPECTS

Care coordination and appointment management

Care coordination and appointment management are essential links in the chain of medical care, particularly in a field as vast and dynamic as dermatology. Whether it's an initial consultation, regular follow-up or specialist treatment, efficient management of these elements ensures not only that processes run smoothly, but also that patients receive better care.

At the heart of the healthcare system, appointments are like the beat of a pulse, marking the rhythm of clinical life. However, managing these appointments is not as simple as ticking a box on a calendar. It involves juggling emergencies, follow-ups, invasive procedures, simple consultations and much more, while taking care to respect the time constraints of both patients and healthcare professionals.

Care coordination, meanwhile, is a complex dance involving multiple stakeholders. In dermatology, this can mean working hand in hand with plastic surgeons, oncologists, allergists, specialist nurses and many other specialists. This coordination is essential to ensure that each patient receives the right care, at the right time, from the right specialist. It's a delicate balancing act, where communication is key.

The advent of modern technology has made it much easier to manage appointments and coordinate care. Electronic patient record management systems provide an overview of medical history, upcoming appointments and current treatments. What's more, with telemedicine on the rise, remote consultations have become a reality, offering unprecedented flexibility.

However, human skills are more important than technology. The ability to listen, understand and anticipate patients' needs is invaluable. Every patient is unique, with his or her own concerns, needs and medical history. Ensuring smooth coordination of care and efficient management of appointments means recognising and respecting this uniqueness.

Care coordination and appointment management are not simply administrative tasks. They are at the heart of the patient experience, directly influencing the quality of care, patient satisfaction and, ultimately, health outcomes. In the complex and ever-changing world of dermatology, these elements play a pivotal role in ensuring that every patient receives timely, appropriate and well-coordinated care.

Financial aspects and insurance

Navigating the tumultuous waters of finance and insurance in the medical sector, and particularly in dermatology, is a challenge that many patients and healthcare professionals encounter. Dermatology, with its wide range of procedures, from medically necessary treatments to elective cosmetic procedures, presents a mosaic of financial considerations that require in-depth understanding and careful management.

The reality is that medical care is expensive. Whether it's routine consultations, surgery or specialist treatment, there's always a cost associated with it. For many, insurance eases this burden, but it brings its own set of complications and details to consider.

The first step for patients is often to understand exactly what their insurance covers. Not all insurance policies are created equal. Some may cover routine dermatology consultations, while others may exclude specific procedures or only partially cover them. In addition, the distinction between "medically necessary" treatments and "cosmetic" or "aesthetic" procedures can often be blurred, leading to unexpected surprises when it comes to billing.

From the point of view of the healthcare professional, mastery of the financial aspects is just as crucial. This involves not only an understanding of operational costs, but also an in-depth knowledge of the different insurance schemes, billing codes and reimbursement procedures. Poor management or lack of knowledge of these elements can lead to late payment, denial of cover or even litigation.

In this complex context, transparency is the key. Patients have the right to know in advance the costs associated with their care. Open communication between patient and healthcare professional, where costs, treatment options and insurance details are clearly discussed, can help avoid future confusion or frustration.

In addition, with the rapidly changing healthcare and insurance landscape, keeping up to date with the latest trends, regulations and options available is essential. Healthcare professionals can consider specific training or workshops to keep up to date, while patients can benefit from educational resources or consultations with financial specialists or insurance advisors.

Although the financial and insurance aspects of dermatology can seem daunting, with thorough understanding, transparent communication and proactive management, they can be successfully navigated. After all, the ultimate goal is to ensure that patients receive the best possible care, regardless of financial challenges.

Supplies management, equipment and medicines

Managing supplies, equipment and medicines is a crucial part of the day-to-day running of any dermatology unit. Whether it's a large hospital clinic, a small private practice or a research centre, the efficiency with which these elements are managed can greatly influence the quality of care, productivity and even patient safety.

In the field of dermatology, the diversity of procedures and treatments requires a wide range of supplies, specialist equipment and medicines. This diversity, while enabling personalised and effective medical care, also requires meticulous management to ensure continuity of care.

Supplies include everything from gloves and bandages to specific surgical instruments. Managing them requires regular stock-taking to ensure that there are no stock-outs, especially for frequently used items. Regular quality checks are also essential to ensure that supplies remain sterile and in good condition.

Dermatology **equipment** can be as basic as a magnifying lamp or as advanced as a phototherapy device or dermatological laser. Preventive maintenance is crucial here. Faulty or poorly calibrated equipment can not only compromise care but also present a risk to the patient. What's more, as technology advances, it's important to keep abreast of the latest innovations and, where necessary, consider upgrades or replacements.

Medicines used in dermatology range from topical creams to advanced biological agents. Managing medicines involves ensuring that they are stored correctly, do not exceed their expiry date and are dispensed accurately. With the constant emergence of new drugs and therapies, ongoing training for staff is often necessary to ensure safe and effective use.

Beyond simple stock management, there is the issue of coordination with suppliers and manufacturers. Establishing solid relationships with these stakeholders can facilitate ordering, delivery and even price negotiation.

Another crucial aspect is staff training and awareness. Every member of the team must be aware of the importance of proper resource management and know how to use and maintain supplies and equipment correctly.

Effective management of supplies, equipment and medicines in dermatology is not just a question of operational efficiency. It is an essential element in ensuring quality of care, patient safety and staff satisfaction. In the fast pace of modern medicine, these details may seem minor, but their impact on the patient and the healthcare system as a whole is anything but negligible.

Chapter 16: DERMATOLOGY AND SYSTEMIC PATHOLOGIES

Skin manifestations internal illnesses

The cutaneous manifestations of internal illnesses illustrate the complexity of the human body and the way in which its different systems are inextricably linked. The skin, often described as a mirror of the body's general state, can reflect imbalances or problems occurring in distant parts of the body. These dermatological manifestations can be the first indication of an internal illness, sometimes a serious one, requiring medical intervention.

Autoimmune diseases such as systemic lupus erythematosus can cause malar or discoid eruptions. Dermatomyositis, on the other hand, often manifests itself as purplish skin eruptions on the eyelids and rough patches on the joints.
Liver disease can lead to a number of skin manifestations. Cirrhosis, for example, can cause "spider veins" (telangiectasias), jaundice or pruritus. Similarly, haemochromatosis, an iron overload, can give the skin a bronze tint.
Kidney disease, particularly renal failure, can lead to paleness due to anaemia, pale yellow discolouration or xerosis (dry skin).
Endocrine imbalances also play a role in skin manifestations. Myxedema, due to hypothyroidism, results in dry, cold, oedematous skin. Hyperthyroidism, on the other hand, can result in warm, moist skin. Diabetes mellitus can cause skin infections, diabetic ulcers or eruptive xanthomas.

Lung conditions such as cyanosis, due to heart or lung failure, manifest themselves as bluish discolouration of the skin, particularly around the lips and nails.
Gastrointestinal diseases, such as coeliac disease, can lead to symptoms such as dermatitis herpetiformis, characterised by intense, itchy blisters, usually on the elbows, knees and buttocks.
Infections such as secondary syphilis can cause rashes on the palms of the hands and soles of the feet, while infective endocarditis can cause Osler nodules or Janeway spots.
Early detection of these skin manifestations can be key to diagnosing the underlying internal disease. This requires an interdisciplinary approach to medicine, where dermatologists work closely with other specialists to ensure comprehensive patient care. Understanding the interconnections between the skin and the internal organs is essential to effective medical practice, as it enables us to look beyond isolated symptoms and understand the patient as a whole.

The nurse and illness autoimmune with dermatological manifestations

The nurse dealing with autoimmune diseases with dermatological manifestations is often the first healthcare professional to interact closely with the patient at different stages of the disease. These diseases, in which the body's immune system attacks its own tissues, can cause a variety of dermatological symptoms, ranging from mild rashes to severe, debilitating lesions.

First signs and diagnosis
During initial consultations, nurses must listen to patients' concerns and be able to identify the typical skin

manifestations of autoimmune diseases. Symptoms vary but may include rashes, red or purplish patches, ulcers or blisters. Careful observation and documentation of these signs help to guide the dermatologist or rheumatologist towards a precise diagnosis.

Patient education
Once the diagnosis has been made, the nurse plays an essential role in patient education. This includes explaining the causes and nature of the disease, the treatments available and how to manage symptoms on a day-to-day basis. The nurse also teaches the patient how to care for their skin at home, including the application of topical medication and the care of open wounds.

Treatment management
The management of autoimmune diseases with dermatological manifestations may require a combination of oral, topical and sometimes injectable medications. Nurses are often responsible for managing these treatments, whether administering injections, monitoring side effects or following up with other specialists.

Psychological support
The skin manifestations of autoimmune diseases can have a significant impact on patients' self-esteem and quality of life. Nurses must therefore be sensitive to patients' emotional needs, offering a listening ear, practical advice and, if necessary, referral to psychological support resources or support groups.

Coordination with other healthcare professionals
Nurses often work closely with a multidisciplinary team. This may include dermatologists, rheumatologists, psychologists, nutritionists and other specialists. Coordination of care between these different professionals is essential to ensure complete and effective patient care.

When it comes to autoimmune diseases with dermatological manifestations, the nurse occupies a central position, acting as a bridge between the patient and the rest of the medical team. The nurse's ability to offer attentive, educational and holistic care is crucial to the patient's overall well-being.

Collaboration with other specialities for integrated monitoring

Collaboration between dermatology nurses and other medical specialities is essential to provide integrated, holistic care for patients. This multi-disciplinary approach provides comprehensive care, ensuring that all aspects of a patient's health are considered and treated appropriately.

Exchange of information
Fluid communication between the dermatology nurse and other healthcare professionals is the key to understanding the full range of patient issues. The regular exchange of medical reports, observations and recommendations between specialists ensures that everyone has the most up-to-date information.

Multidisciplinary meetings
Organising regular meetings between the different medical specialities involved in the care of a specific patient enables a coherent care plan to be drawn up. These meetings provide an opportunity to discuss the patient's progress and treatment adjustments, and to ensure that all aspects of the patient's health are taken into account.

Orientation towards other specialities
The dermatology nurse must be well informed about the skills and expertise of other specialists. In this way, when underlying or concomitant health problems are identified, rapid referral to the appropriate specialist can be implemented.

Patient education
Nurses also play an essential role in educating patients about how the various medical specialities interact for their

well-being. By understanding the role of each specialist and how they work together, patients can better engage in their own care process.

Continuing education

To ensure effective collaboration, it is important for dermatology nurses to take part in ongoing training, not only in their specific field but also in related areas. This enables them to keep abreast of the latest advances in other specialities and improve the coordination of care.

Special cases: systemic diseases

In the case of diseases with skin manifestations but also other systemic symptoms, collaboration is all the more crucial. For example, lupus can affect not only the skin, but also the kidneys, heart and lungs. In such cases, the dermatology nurse must work closely with nephrologists, cardiologists, pulmonologists and other specialists to ensure comprehensive care.

Collaboration between the dermatology nurse and other specialties is essential to provide integrated and comprehensive care for patients. It requires open communication, ongoing training and a commitment to the patient's overall well-being.

Chapter 17: SKIN INFECTIONS AND TROPICAL DISEASES

Recognition common and rare infections

Recognising and effectively treating skin infections, whether common or rare, is essential to the role of a dermatology nurse. Skin infections can be bacterial, viral, fungal or parasitic in origin, and their management varies according to their nature and severity.

Common infections
- **Impetigo**: Superficial bacterial infection often caused by staphylococcus or streptococcus, in the form of oozing red patches which develop into golden crusts.
- **Boils and carbuncles**: These deep purulent infections are caused mainly by staphylococcus aureus. They take the form of painful abscesses.
- **Skin mycoses**: These are caused by fungi. The areas most commonly affected are the feet (athlete's foot), groin (Hebra's marginal eczema) and scalp.
- **Warts**: Caused by the human papillomavirus (HPV), these are contagious and can appear on any part of the body.
- **Herpes**: This viral infection is characterised by painful blisters, mainly on the lips (herpes labialis) or genitals.

Rare infections
- **Syphilis**: This sexually transmitted disease caused by the *Treponema pallidum* bacterium can lead to specific skin lesions in its various stages.
- **Cutaneous leishmaniasis**: caused by a parasite transmitted by the bite of a sandfly, it causes skin ulcers that heal slowly.

Sporotrichosis: Deep fungal infection that can cause nodules and ulcerations along the lymphatic tract.

Pian: A tropical disease caused by the bacterium *Treponema pertenue*, it manifests itself as nodules and ulcers.

For each infection, the dermatology nurse must know the specific signs and symptoms, the appropriate diagnostic methods and the recommended treatments. In addition, it is crucial to educate patients about prevention, particularly for contagious infections.

Nurses also need to keep abreast of new research and therapeutic advances in the field of skin infections, as pathogens evolve and new strains may emerge, requiring appropriate treatment approaches.

Approach to skin diseases linked to travel and geography

The influence of travel and geography on skin health is both a fascinating and essential topic for dermatology nursing practice. With globalisation and the increasing number of people travelling from one continent to another, skin diseases that were once confined to specific regions are now being found in areas where they were previously unknown.

The influence of climate

Dry and desert climates: These areas can lead to skin dehydration, sunburn, cracks and even lesions caused by wind and sand.

Humid and tropical climates: These regions are prone to fungal infections such as ringworm or athlete's foot, and parasitic infections such as leishmaniasis or scabies.

Endemic diseases by region

- **Africa**: Diseases such as yaws, trypanosomiasis (sleeping sickness) and various forms of leishmaniasis.
- **Asia**: In addition to certain specific fungal and bacterial infections, leprosy, although increasingly rare, is still present in certain regions.
- **South and Central America**: Some regions are home to diseases such as leishmaniasis, Chagas disease and other parasitic infections.
- **Oceania**: In certain regions of the Pacific, diseases such as lymphatic filariasis can cause skin disorders.

Precautions for travellers

- **Vaccinations** : Before travelling, it is essential to find out about the vaccinations needed to prevent certain cutaneous or systemic diseases with skin manifestations.
- **Protection against insects**: In many regions, mosquitoes, ticks and other insects can transmit skin diseases. The use of repellents and mosquito nets is recommended.
- **Hygiene advice**: Travellers should be informed of the importance of maintaining good hygiene, washing clothes regularly and protecting themselves from direct exposure to fresh water in certain regions at risk of schistosomiasis, for example.

Continuing education and up-to-date knowledge of travel-related skin diseases are essential for dermatology nurses. Not only does this enable them to make a correct diagnosis, but it also helps them to advise patients effectively before and after their travels, thereby ensuring better skin health and disease prevention.

Prevention and advice for travellers

Travelling is an enriching experience that opens up horizons and encourages the discovery of new cultures. However, it is essential to take certain precautions to protect your health, particularly that of your skin. Dermatology nurses, armed with their expertise, play a crucial role in raising awareness and preparing travellers.

1. Pre-departure preparation
   Medical consultation: It is advisable to consult a doctor or vaccination centre several weeks before departure. Some vaccines require several doses spaced out or a certain period of time to be effective.
   First-aid kit: A kit adapted to the destination, including antiseptics, dressings, sun creams, mosquito repellents and possibly antifungals or antiparasitics, is essential.
2. Protection from the sun
   Sun cream: Choose a broad-spectrum sun cream with a high protection factor that is water-resistant, and reapply every two hours and after every swim.
   Appropriate clothing: Light, long, natural-fibre clothing can protect against UV rays. Wide-brimmed hats and sunglasses are also essential.
   Avoid peak times: The sun is strongest between 10 am and 4 pm. If possible, stay in the shade during these hours.
3. Protection against insects
   Repellents: Use repellents on exposed skin and clothing. Some repellents can be applied directly to clothing for extra protection.
   Mosquito nets: If you sleep in an area where mosquitoes are active, an insecticide-treated mosquito net is essential.

4. Food and hygiene precautions
    - **Drinking water**: Drink sealed bottled water. Avoid ice cubes in drinks.
    - **Food**: Make sure food is well cooked and eaten hot. Avoid unpeeled fruit and vegetables.
    - **Hand hygiene**: Wash your hands regularly, especially before eating. Use an alcohol-based hand sanitiser if soap and water are not available.
5. Recognition of risks specific to the region
    - **Get the facts**: Every destination has its own risks. Whether it's endemic diseases, local parasites or environmental problems, a good knowledge of local risks is essential.
    - **Stay informed**: Regularly check updates on health risks associated with your destination.

With these preventive measures, travellers can make the most of their trip while protecting their health and that of their skin. The dermatology nurse's expert advice helps to make every journey safer and more enjoyable.

Chapter 18:
DERMATOLOGY IN SPECIFIC CONTEXTS

Dermatology in hospitals versus private practice

Dermatology, like many other medical specialities, can be practised in a variety of settings. While some dermatologists choose to work in hospitals or medical centres, others prefer the independent nature of a private practice. Each of these settings offers unique advantages and disadvantages that can influence how a dermatologist practices and cares for their patients.

1. Working environment

    Hospital: In the hospital setting, the dermatologist generally works closely with other specialists. Access to state-of-the-art equipment is often easier, and the cases encountered can be more diverse, particularly because of emergencies or patients admitted to hospital with co-morbidities.

    Private practice: In a private practice, the dermatologist is generally the main decision-maker. They can shape their working environment to suit their preferences, choose their staff and decide what equipment to acquire. The patient-practitioner relationship can also be more personal.

2. Types of cases handled

    Hospital: Cases are often more complex, and the dermatologist may be called in for emergency consultations, pathologies associated with other medical conditions, or surgical procedures requiring hospitalisation.

- **Private practice**: While private dermatologists can also treat complex cases, they are likely to see more patients for regular check-ups, cosmetic consultations or common skin conditions.
3. Professional autonomy
    - **Hospital**: Although dermatologists make independent medical decisions, they often have to comply with hospital procedures and protocols, collaborate with other departments and adapt to the hospital infrastructure.
    - **Private practice**: Dermatologists in private practice enjoy considerable autonomy in managing their practice, selecting their staff and establishing their own protocols.
4. Financial aspects
    - **Hospital**: In a hospital environment, the salary is often fixed or based on a contract, offering a degree of financial security.
    - **Private practice**: While the income potential may be higher in private practice, it is also associated with greater responsibilities, particularly in terms of management, rents, equipment purchases and insurance.
5. Continuing education and research
    - **Hospital**: Hospitals, especially those affiliated to university institutions, often offer more opportunities for research, teaching and continuing education.
    - **Private practice**: Although continuing education is always a priority, dermatologists in private practice often have to take the initiative to continue their training and participate actively in it.

The choice between a hospital setting and a private practice depends on each dermatologist's professional aspirations, personal preferences and circumstances. Each environment has its own challenges and rewards, but both allow the practitioner to provide essential care to those who need it.

Dermatology in rural versus urban areas

Dermatology is an essential speciality for the health of the skin, hair and nails. But depending on the environment in which it is practised, whether rural or urban, the challenges and opportunities can vary considerably. Let's delve into these two worlds and explore the nuances of each environment.

1. Access to care and density of services

    Rural areas: In rural areas, access to specialists, including dermatologists, may be limited. A single dermatologist may serve a large geographical area, which can make appointments less accessible for patients in remote areas. This could lead to longer waiting times or significant travel for patients.

    Urban areas: Urban areas, with a higher population density, tend to have several dermatologists, sometimes even in the same neighbourhood. This can make it easier for patients to access care.

2. Specialisation and diversity of cases

    Rural environment: With the potential to be one of the few dermatologists in the region, the professional may be called upon to treat a wide range of cases, from common ailments to rarer cases.

    Urban environment: With a greater concentration of specialists, you may see more sub-specialisations (such as paediatric or cosmetic dermatology) and clinics dedicated to certain conditions.

3. Collaboration and resources

    Rural environment: Direct collaboration with other specialists may be limited by distance, although telemedicine can facilitate these interactions. State-of-the-art resources and equipment may also be less accessible.

Urban environment: The proximity of hospitals, research centres and other specialists facilitates direct collaboration and rapid access to new technologies and treatments.

4. Patient knowledge and community approach

Rural environment: Working in a rural area can offer a closer bond with patients. Dermatologists can get to know their patients and their families over several generations, offering a more holistic approach.

Urban environment: If the volume of patients is higher, the relationship can become more clinical, although it is still possible to build strong links.

5. Financial and career issues

Rural areas: Although there may be less competition, income may be moderated by patient volume. However, certain government initiatives sometimes encourage specialists to practice in rural areas through financial incentives.

Urban environment: While revenue potential may be high due to patient volume, competition is also stronger.

Whether in a rural or urban environment, the role of the dermatologist is vital. Each environment presents its own challenges and opportunities. The choice depends on the aspirations, values and personal priorities of the professional.

Dermatological care in emergency or disaster situations

In critical times, when urgency and disaster reign, dermatology may not be the first medical field that springs to mind. However, skin health is an essential aspect of general well-being, particularly in crisis situations where external conditions can have a direct and serious impact on the epidermis.

1. Recognising skin emergencies:
In times of disaster, professionals need to be able to quickly distinguish between benign skin conditions and dermatological emergencies that require immediate intervention. Conditions such as necrotising fasciitis, a rapid and fatal infection, must be treated without delay.

2. Burns and trauma:
Disasters, whether fires, explosions or armed conflicts, can result in serious burns. Initial care, assessment of severity, decontamination and treatment of burns are crucial to preventing complications.

3. Exposure-related illnesses:
In the context of natural disasters such as floods, hurricanes or earthquakes, individuals may be exposed to stagnant water, debris or other conditions conducive to skin infections. Bacterial, fungal or parasitic infections can occur.

4. Stress-related rashes and psychological trauma:
Traumatic events can trigger or aggravate certain skin conditions, such as psoriasis or eczema. Taking the psychological aspect into account is essential for comprehensive treatment.

5. Hygiene conditions and propagation:
In emergency situations, particularly in refugee camps or disaster areas, hygiene can be compromised, facilitating the spread of contagious skin diseases such as scabies or fungal infections.

6. Exposure to chemical or biological agents:
In the event of a chemical attack or accidental spillage of hazardous substances, the skin is often the first organ to be affected. Rapid decontamination and treatment of skin lesions are essential.

7. Supply and logistics:
In crisis zones, access to essential medicines and equipment may be limited. Preparing for such situations requires solid logistics to ensure the supply of necessary resources, such as antibiotic creams, antiseptics and dressings.

8. Training and preparation:
Training health professionals in emergency dermatological care is essential. Regular simulations and exercises can help prepare teams to act quickly and effectively in the event of a disaster.

Although dermatology is not always at the forefront of an emergency or disaster, skin health remains essential. Preparation, early recognition of conditions and appropriate intervention can save lives and prevent long-term complications. At such times, the role of the dermatologist, in collaboration with other specialists, is invaluable.

Chapter 19:
LEGAL ASPECTS IN DERMATOLOGY

Informed consent and invasive procedures

Informed consent is a fundamental pillar of modern medicine, based on respect for the autonomy and dignity of the patient. When it comes to invasive procedures, particularly in dermatology, this consent takes on vital importance in ensuring that the patient is fully aware of the risks, benefits and alternatives available.

1. The philosophy of informed consent :
The concept is based on the idea that each individual has the inalienable right to decide what is done to their body. The role of the healthcare professional is to educate, inform and guide, but never to coerce.

2. The essential elements of consent :

Information: Before any procedure, the patient must be informed of the relevant details, including the nature of the operation, the associated risks, the expected benefits and possible alternatives.

Understanding: Providing information is not enough; the professional must ensure that the patient fully understands the implications.

Willingness: Consent must be given freely, without external or internal pressure.

3. Common invasive procedures in dermatology :
These procedures can range from simple skin biopsies to more complex surgical interventions, such as melanoma excision or reconstructive surgery.

4. Specific risks :
Each procedure has its own risks. For example, a biopsy may result in bleeding, infection or scarring, while more extensive procedures may have anaesthetic complications or prolonged recovery times.

5. Expected benefits :
As well as diagnosing or treating the disease, there may be psychological benefits, such as relieving the anxiety associated with a suspected lesion.

6. Alternatives :
For some conditions, other treatment options may be available, including other types of surgery, drug therapies or monitoring.

7. Documentation :
Properly obtained informed consent must be documented, often in the form of a signed form. This document protects both the patient and the healthcare professional.

8. Special situations :
There may be times when the patient is unable to give consent, such as in a medical emergency, mental incapacity or when the patient is a minor. In these situations, the healthcare professional will need to navigate delicately, seeking the consent of legal guardians or acting in the patient's best interests.

The relationship between the healthcare professional and the patient is based on trust. The informed consent process reinforces this trust, ensuring that the patient is an active and informed partner in decisions concerning his or her health. In dermatology, as in all branches of medicine, respecting patient autonomy by obtaining informed consent is both an ethical and a legal obligation.

Managing complications and medical errors

Complications and medical errors, although inevitable, are delicate and difficult aspects of medical practice. In dermatology, as in other specialities, it is crucial to manage them with sensitivity, honesty and professionalism.

1. Recognising complications and errors :
The first step in managing problems properly is to recognise them. This may mean monitoring post-operative symptoms, re-evaluating biopsy results, or admitting an error in prescribing medication.

2. Inform the patient immediately:
Honesty is essential. If a complication has arisen or an error has been made, it is the duty of the healthcare professional to inform the patient in a transparent and comprehensible manner.

3. Listening and empathy :
It is essential to provide a space where patients can express their concerns, frustrations or fears. Empathy, active listening and support are crucial to rebuilding trust.

4. Finding a solution :
When an error occurs, the healthcare professional must immediately look for ways to correct it, whether this means additional treatment, referral to a specialist, or another intervention.

5. Avoid defensiveness :
It is natural to want to protect oneself or rationalise mistakes. However, it is essential to remain open and honest, and to put the patient's well-being first.

6. Analysis and prevention :
After the immediate management of the complication or error, it is crucial to analyse what happened. This may include a case review with colleagues, an update of protocols or additional training. The aim is to prevent such incidents from happening again.

7. Legal aspects :
Medical errors can have legal implications. It is essential to be well informed about rights and responsibilities, and to consult with legal advisers if necessary. Accurate and transparent documentation is crucial.

8. Support for healthcare professionals :
Medical errors can have an emotional impact on healthcare professionals themselves. Seeking support, whether through colleagues, mentors or professional therapy, can be essential in managing the associated stress and guilt.

Medical complications and errors, while regrettable, offer opportunities for learning and improvement. By managing these incidents with honesty, integrity and empathy, healthcare professionals can not only mitigate the consequences for the patient, but also strengthen trust and understanding between patient and carer. The key is to always put the patient's needs and well-being first.

Patients' rights and professional responsibilities

In the medical field, patient rights and professional responsibilities are two sides of the same coin, intertwining closely to ensure high-quality, ethical and respectful care. Here is a fluid exploration of this essential interplay, particularly in dermatology.

Patients' fundamental rights :

Right to information: Every patient has the right to be informed in a clear and comprehensible manner about his or her state of health, the proposed treatments, their benefits and risks, and possible alternatives.

Informed consent: Before any intervention or treatment, patients must give their consent after having been properly informed.

Right to confidentiality: A patient's medical information is private. It should only be shared with the healthcare professionals involved in the patient's care, unless there is explicit consent or a legal obligation to do so.

Right to respect and dignity: Every patient must be treated with respect, whatever their race, religion, origin, socio-economic situation or medical condition.

Right of access to medical records: Patients may ask to consult or obtain a copy of their medical records.

Right to refuse treatment: Even after being informed of the consequences, a patient may refuse treatment or an intervention.

Professional responsibilities :

Duty to inform: The healthcare professional has a responsibility to inform the patient fully, clearly and impartially.

Respecting informed consent: Healthcare professionals must ensure that patients have fully understood the information provided and that they have given their informed consent.

Competence and up-to-date knowledge: Caregivers must guarantee ongoing training, in order to offer the best possible care based on the latest medical advances.

Effective communication: Clear communication with the patient, but also with other members of the care team, is essential to ensure coordinated and effective care.

Confidentiality: Healthcare professionals must take all necessary precautions to protect their patients' medical information.

- **Ethics and integrity**: The decisions and actions of healthcare professionals must always be guided by medical ethics, always putting the patient's well-being first.

The balance between patients' rights and professional responsibilities is fundamental to guaranteeing quality dermatological care. By being informed and respected, patients become active players in their own health, while professionals, by respecting their responsibilities, ensure care based on trust, respect and excellence.

Chapter 20:
DERMATOLOGY AND VULNERABLE POPULATIONS

Dermatological care for the elderly

As we age, our skin undergoes changes that require specific attention and care. The effects of time, combined with years of exposure to the elements, can lead to a variety of dermatological concerns in the elderly. This section takes an in-depth look at dermatological care for this age group, highlighting its specific features.

1. Age-related skin changes :
   Reduced elasticity: Over time, the skin loses its elasticity, leading to the formation of wrinkles and sagging.
   Increased dryness: Sebum production decreases with age, making skin drier and more prone to flaking and itching.
   Changes in pigmentation: Years of sun exposure can lead to brown spots (solar lentigos) or depigmented areas.
   Increased sensitivity: Thin, dry skin is more susceptible to injury, and also takes longer to heal.
2. Common skin conditions in the elderly :
   Seborrhoeic and actinic keratoses: These benign lesions may be rough to the touch and vary in colour from pink to brown.
   Carcinomas: Years of sun exposure increase the risk of basal and squamous cell carcinomas.
   Varicosities: These small, dilated veins are common on the legs.

- **Atrophy**: Thinning of the skin, making it translucent and fragile.

3. Principles of skin care for mature skin :
- **Moisturising**: Daily use of moisturising creams and lotions helps maintain the skin barrier.
- **Sun protection**: Even at an advanced age, it is essential to protect the skin from the harmful effects of UV rays.
- **Topical treatments**: Certain medications can help treat specific age-related skin conditions.
- **Regular check-ups**: Regular visits to the dermatologist are essential to monitor and treat any skin anomalies.

4. Psychological issues :
Skin changes can have an impact on self-esteem and body image. It is therefore crucial to address these concerns and offer appropriate support.

5. Interprofessional collaboration :
Treating the elderly often requires collaboration between dermatologists, general practitioners, geriatricians and other specialists to ensure a comprehensive approach.

Geriatric dermatology requires an attentive and personalised approach, taking into account the unique challenges faced by the elderly. By combining medical science, compassion and listening, it is possible to offer the elderly the skin care they need while respecting their dignity and overall well-being.

Dermatology and immunocompromised patients

The management of immunocompromised patients in dermatology is complex and requires a thorough understanding of the specific challenges associated with this population. Because of their weakened immune systems, these patients are more likely to develop skin conditions that may be atypical, severe or resistant to standard treatments.

1. Background to immunodepression :
    Definition and types : Immunosuppression is a reduction in the immune system's ability to fight infections and other diseases. It can be caused by diseases (such as HIV), drugs (immunosuppressants, chemotherapy) or other causes (organ transplants, for example).
2. Common skin conditions in immunocompromised patients :
    Opportunistic infections: Because of their weakened immune systems, these patients are more likely to contract skin infections caused by bacteria, viruses, fungi or parasites.
    Skin tumours: Certain skin cancers are more common and may be more aggressive in immunocompromised patients.
    Skin manifestations of systemic diseases: Diseases such as HIV can present specific dermatological signs.
3. Diagnosis and monitoring :
    Clinical examination: It is essential to carry out regular skin examinations to identify and treat any abnormalities quickly.
    Diagnostic tests: Biopsies, cultures and other tests may be required to diagnose skin disorders in these patients.
4. Therapeutic management :
    Topical treatments: Medicines applied directly to the skin, such as antifungals or antivirals, can be effective.
    Systemic therapies: In some cases, oral or injectable medical intervention may be necessary.

- **Special precautions**: Due to their immunocompromised state, some medicines may have increased side effects for these patients.
5. The importance of prevention :
   - **Avoiding triggers**: It is crucial for immunocompromised patients to avoid situations that could aggravate their condition, such as excessive exposure to the sun or contact with sick people.
   - **Vaccinations**: Although some vaccinations may be contraindicated for certain immunocompromised patients, others are essential to prevent serious illnesses.
6. Interprofessional collaboration :

The management of immunocompromised patients often requires close collaboration between dermatologists, infectiologists, oncologists and other specialists to ensure comprehensive care.

Immunocompromised patients present unique challenges in dermatology, requiring specific vigilance and expertise. A holistic, patient-centred approach, combined with interdisciplinary collaboration, can help to improve the quality of life of these patients while effectively managing their skin conditions.

Skin care for patients at the end of life

When a person is terminally ill, the quality of the care they receive becomes all the more crucial. Skin care for patients at the end of life is not just a question of aesthetics or comfort, but plays a major role in ensuring the patient's respect and dignity.

1. Understanding the issues:
   Physiological changes: At the end of life, the skin can become thinner, drier and less elastic. It is also more susceptible to injury and infection.
   Associated symptoms: Dehydration, reduced mobility, medication, and other factors can contribute to skin problems.
2. Pressure sores and lesions:
   Prevention: Regular patient rotation, the use of special cushions and good hygiene are crucial.
   Treatment: The management of pressure sores requires regular assessment, appropriate cleansing, and sometimes topical treatments.
3. Care for dry, delicate skin:
   Moisturising: Applying creams and ointments regularly can help maintain the skin's integrity.
   Gentle baths: Warm baths with mild products can help to clean without irritating.
4. Management of skin infections:
   Early recognition: Early detection of signs of infection allows rapid intervention.
   Appropriate treatment: This may include topical or oral antibiotics.
5. Comfort and pain relief:
   Soothing gels and creams: Some products can provide temporary relief from itching or pain.
   Medication: Analgesics may be required to treat pain associated with severe skin conditions.
6. Psychosocial care:
   Dignity and respect: Maintaining the cleanliness and integrity of patients' skin helps to preserve their dignity.
   Communication: Discuss skin needs and concerns openly with patients and their families.

7. Working with the care team:
- **Care coordination**: Working closely with doctors, nurses, Caregivers and other specialists to ensure comprehensive care.
- **Education**: Training nursing staff in best practice in skin care for patients at the end of life.

Skin care for patients at the end of life is an essential aspect of palliative care. It requires meticulous attention, clinical expertise and a compassionate approach. By focusing on the patient's comfort, dignity and well-being, healthcare professionals can offer invaluable support during this delicate period.

Chapter 21:
PAIN MANAGEMENT AND SYMPTOMS

Dealing with chronic pain linked to skin conditions

Skin pain, often perceived as a minor symptom compared with other forms of chronic pain, is nonetheless a very real and sometimes debilitating reality for patients suffering from skin disorders. It interacts in complex ways with the patient's physiology, psychology and general well-being.

1. The reality of skin pain:
   Multidimensional nature: Skin pain can be acute, chronic, stabbing, burning or itching. It varies in intensity and can be continuous or intermittent.
   Various origins: It can result from inflammation, infection, nerve damage or vascular disorders.
2. Impact on quality of life:
   Sleep disturbances: Pain or itching can disrupt the sleep cycle, leading to fatigue and mood disorders.
   Everyday difficulties: Simple activities such as showering, dressing or even sitting down can become painful.
   Psychological effects: Chronic pain can lead to anxiety, depression and social isolation.
3. Pain assessment:
   Pain scales: Using standardised tools to quantify pain and its progression.
   Pain diary: Encourage patients to keep a diary detailing the nature, intensity and duration of their pain.

4. Therapeutic approaches:
    - **Topical treatments:** analgesic or anti-inflammatory creams, ointments and gels.
    - **Oral medication:** analgesics, anti-inflammatories, antihistamines or even anticonvulsants for neuropathic pain.
    - **Alternative therapies**: Acupuncture, cold/heat or light therapy.
5. Psychological support:
    - **Cognitive-behavioural therapy (CBT):** helping patients to manage their pain and associated emotions.
    - **Support group**: Share and exchange with other patients going through similar experiences.
6. Education and prevention:
    - **Avoiding triggers**: Identifying and avoiding aggravating factors, whether environmental, chemical or other.
    - **Skin care**: An appropriate skin care routine to protect the skin and prevent the pain from worsening.
7. Interprofessional collaboration:
    - **Multidisciplinary team**: Dermatologists, nurses, neurologists, psychologists and other specialists can work together to provide holistic pain management.

Tackling chronic pain linked to skin disorders requires a multidimensional, personalised approach. By placing the patient at the heart of the treatment and integrating medical, psychological and educational solutions, it is possible to manage this pain more effectively and significantly improve patients' quality of life.

Palliative care in dermatology

When we think of palliative care, we often think of serious conditions such as cancer, heart disease or dementia.

However, palliative care in dermatology is just as crucial, although less recognised. It focuses on alleviating symptoms and improving quality of life for patients with advanced or incurable dermatological diseases.

1. The need for palliative care in dermatology :
   Complexity of symptoms: Dermatological conditions, although they may appear superficial, can lead to intense pain, itching, infection and psychological complications.
   Impact on quality of life: Skin manifestations can profoundly alter patients' self-esteem, social interaction and daily functional capacity.
2. Common symptoms and their management :
   Pain: Use of topical analgesics, anti-inflammatories or other drugs for neuropathic pain.
   Pruritus: Skin hydration, antihistamines, phototherapy or systemic treatments may be used.
   Impaired skin integrity: dressings, antibacterial creams and wound care.
3. Psychosocial approach :
   Psychological support: Therapy, counselling and support groups to help patients manage the emotional impact of skin diseases.
   Communication: Providing clear and honest information about the disease and its prognosis, while listening and responding to patients' concerns.
4. Collaboration with other specialities :
   Multidisciplinary team: Dermatologists, nurses, psychologists, social workers and other health professionals work together to meet patients' complex needs.
5. Spiritual and cultural aspects :
   Respect for beliefs: Understanding and respecting patients' spiritual and cultural beliefs in order to provide patient-centred care.

- **Rituals and customs**: Facilitating the practice of rituals and customs that can help patients find comfort and meaning.
6. End-of-life decision :
    - **Anticipatory discussions**: conversations about the patient's wishes and preferences for the end of life, including advance directives and decisions about resuscitation.
    - **Symptom management**: Ensuring patient comfort, reducing pain and other disturbing symptoms.

Palliative care in dermatology is an essential facet of patient-centred care. It requires a holistic approach that takes into account not only the physical symptoms, but also the emotional, social and spiritual needs of patients. By recognising and responding to these needs, healthcare professionals can offer compassionate and dignified quality care to those facing advanced or incurable dermatological disease.

Non-pharmacological strategies for managing pain and pruritus

Pain and pruritus, or itching, are two symptoms frequently associated with a variety of dermatological conditions. Although pharmacological interventions are often preferred, non-pharmacological methods can play a crucial role as a complement to drug treatments, or for those seeking less invasive alternatives. These approaches can not only relieve these symptoms, but also improve patients' overall quality of life.

1. Behavioural measures :
    - **Cognitive-behavioural therapy (CBT)**: CBT helps to identify and change the negative thoughts and behaviours associated with pain and pruritus,

teaching patients strategies to manage their symptoms.

Biofeedback: This method teaches patients to control certain bodily functions to help reduce pain or itching.

2. Relaxation techniques :

    Deep breathing: Breathing in deeply, then exhaling slowly, can help relax the body and divert attention from the pain.

    Guided visualisation: Imagining a peaceful place or scene can have a calming effect.

    Meditation and mindfulness: Focusing attention on the present moment can help reduce stress and minimise the perception of pain.

3. Physical intervention :

    Thermotherapy: The use of heat, such as hot compresses, can soothe certain types of skin pain.

    Cryotherapy: In certain cases, cold, such as cold compresses, can be beneficial.

    Massage: Massage can improve circulation, reduce stress and relieve muscle tension, which can help reduce pain.

4. Electrical stimulation :

    Transcutaneous electrical nerve stimulation (TENS): This method uses small electrical currents to stimulate the nerves and reduce pain.

5. Complementary approaches :

    Acupuncture: This ancient Chinese technique, which involves inserting fine needles into the skin at specific points, can be effective in treating pain and itching.

    Aromatherapy: Certain essential oils may have soothing or anti-inflammatory properties.

    Herbal therapies: Herbal remedies such as aloe vera or chamomile can soothe irritated skin.

6. Lifestyle changes :

    Oatmeal baths: Colloidal oatmeal has soothing properties that can help reduce itching.

- **Moisturising the skin**: Use emollients or moisturisers regularly to keep the skin hydrated and protected.
- **Avoiding triggers**: Identify and avoid substances or conditions that exacerbate pain or itching, such as certain fabrics, detergents or allergens.

Non-pharmacological methods of managing pain and pruritus can offer significant relief without the potential side effects of medication. Although it is essential to consult a healthcare professional for any concerns or persistent symptoms, integrating these approaches can significantly improve patients' well-being.

Chapter 22:
PSYCHODERMATOLOGICAL ASPECTS

The interface between psychology and dermatology

The interface between psychology and dermatology is a fascinating intersection of mind and body, illustrating the extent to which our skin and psyche are inextricably linked. The skin, as the outermost organ, is often the site of visible manifestations of internal disorders, both physical and psychological. It reflects not only our state of health, but also our emotions, stresses and worries.

Looking at this relationship, it is clear that many dermatological conditions have a significant psychological component. For example, conditions such as psoriasis or eczema can be exacerbated by stress or anxiety. Conversely, living with a visible skin condition can lead to feelings of anxiety, shame or depression, creating a vicious cycle of psychological distress and dermatological symptoms. Rosacea, for example, can be aggravated by embarrassment and stress, but it can also be the cause of these emotions due to the altered appearance of the skin.

Trichotillomania, a disorder in which individuals are driven to pull their hair or pinch their skin, also shows how psychology and dermatology can be closely linked. Here, psychological behaviour leads directly to dermatological trauma.

But this intersection is not limited to illness. The way we perceive our skin and our appearance can have a profound impact on our self-esteem and body image. In an increasingly visual society, perceived imperfections, whether wrinkles, scars or other marks, can have a profound influence on how we see ourselves and how we think others see us.

Recognising this close relationship between the mind and the skin has led to the emergence of 'psychodermatology', a sub-discipline that focuses on the intersection of dermatology and psychology. Psychodermatologists help to treat skin conditions exacerbated by stress or emotions, while also helping patients to manage the psychological distress associated with their skin conditions.

This interface between psychology and dermatology reinforces the idea that to truly heal, we need to adopt a holistic approach. Skin is not only a mirror of our physical state, but also a reflection of our inner world. And for many, the road to healthy skin can start with a healthy understanding and management of the mind.

Management of conditions such as psychogenic pruritus and trichotillomania

The management of conditions at the intersection of dermatology and psychology, such as psychogenic pruritus and trichotillomania, requires a multi-dimensional approach, combining dermatological care and psychological support.

Psychogenic pruritus
Psychogenic pruritus is chronic itching with no apparent dermatological cause, often linked to psychological factors such as stress, anxiety or mood disorders.
Diagnostic approach :
- Exclusion of other causes of itching by dermatological and laboratory tests.

Psychiatric assessment to identify emotional triggers or co-morbidities.

Treatment :

Dermatological care: Emollients can be recommended to reduce skin dryness and antihistamines to manage itching.

Psychological therapies: Cognitive-behavioural therapy can help patients identify and manage itch triggers. Meditation and relaxation techniques can also be useful.

Medication: Antidepressants or anxiolytics may be prescribed if pruritus is associated with depression or anxiety.

Trichotillomania

Trichotillomania, also known as hair-pulling disorder, is a compulsive disorder in which individuals repeatedly pull their hair, resulting in visible alopecia.

Diagnostic approach :

Clinical examination to identify areas of alopecia.

Interviews to understand the seriousness of compulsion.

Treatment :

Cognitive behavioural therapy (CBT): This is the treatment of choice for trichotillomania. CBT helps patients to identify the situations or emotions that trigger the urge to pull their hair and to develop strategies to resist this urge.

Medication: Although there is no specific medication for trichotillomania, some antidepressants or antipsychotics can help reduce symptoms.

Support and education: Support groups can offer invaluable help, enabling patients to share their experiences and learn new coping strategies.

In both cases, close collaboration between dermatologists and mental health professionals is essential. This ensures a holistic approach to treatment, addressing both the skin symptoms and the underlying psychological causes.

The role of the nurse in the management of psychodermatological disorders

In the vast world of dermatology, the intersection between skin diseases and psychological factors has opened the door to a fascinating field called psychodermatology. Here, skin symptoms can often mirror the mind, reflecting internal conflicts, stresses or anxieties. It is in this complex, multi-dimensional context that the role of the nurse takes on its full importance.

Firstly, nurses play a crucial role in the early identification of psychodermatological disorders. Thanks to their regular and often prolonged interaction with patients, nurses can pick up on subtle signs that the patient might not reveal during a brief medical examination. These may include observations of compulsive scratching habits, the presence of self-inflicted lesions or even signs of anxiety or distress when discussing certain skin conditions.

As well as detection, nurses offer emotional support to patients. Recognising and accepting the psychological nature of a skin condition can be difficult for many patients. Some may feel shame, guilt or denial. Nurses, with their empathetic approach and active listening, can offer a listening ear, reassuring patients and helping them navigate the process of understanding and accepting their condition.

Education is also an essential aspect of nursing care. They are responsible for teaching patients about their condition, the treatments available and self-help measures. In the case of psychodermatological disorders, this may include relaxation techniques, methods of managing stress or even references to complementary therapies such as meditation or yoga.

The nurse also acts as a crucial link between the dermatologist and other specialists, such as psychologists or psychiatrists. In the treatment of psychodermatological disorders, an integrated approach is often the most beneficial. The nurse can facilitate this collaboration, ensuring that all parties are kept informed of progress, concerns or changes in the patient's condition.

Last but not least, the dermatology nurse plays a preventive role. Through educational sessions, brochures or one-to-one discussions, the nurse can raise patients' awareness of the links between the skin and the mind, encouraging early treatment and recognition of trigger factors.
In the world of psychodermatology, the nurse acts as a pillar of support, an educator, a coordinator and an advocate, ensuring that patients receive holistic care that treats not only the skin, but also the soul.

Chapter 23:
DERMATOLOGY AND GLOBAL HEALTH

The impact of diet and lifestyle on the skin

In our body's vast ecosystem, every element is interconnected. Like a mirror, the skin, our largest organ, often reflects the internal state of our body. The impact of diet and lifestyle on skin health is a complex interaction, influenced by a multitude of factors and mechanisms.

Food: the power of the plate
Our diet plays a central role in the overall health of our skin. The foods we eat provide essential nutrients that influence cell regeneration, inflammation, hydration and protection against external aggressors.

- **Antioxidants**: Foods rich in antioxidants, such as berries, nuts, green leafy vegetables and green tea, help fight free radicals, which can cause oxidative damage to the skin and accelerate skin ageing.
- **Omega-3 fatty acids**: Found in fish, chia seeds and walnuts, they are essential for maintaining the skin's elasticity and hydration.
- **Water**: Adequate hydration is crucial. Drinking enough water helps to maintain skin elasticity and prevent dryness.
- **Inflammatory foods**: A diet rich in sugars, saturated fats and processed foods can increase inflammation, contributing to conditions such as acne, rosacea and dermatitis.

Lifestyle: Habits that speak for themselves
As well as diet, other aspects of lifestyle have a major influence on skin health.

Stress: Chronic stress can trigger an inflammatory response, exacerbating conditions such as psoriasis or eczema. Relaxation and stress management techniques, such as meditation and yoga, can have beneficial effects.

Sleep: A good night's sleep allows the skin to regenerate itself. Lack of sleep can lead to dark circles, dull skin and increased signs of ageing.

Exercise: Physical activity stimulates blood circulation, which helps to nourish skin cells and eliminate waste products.

Exposure to the sun: Although the sun provides vitamin D, excessive exposure without adequate protection can lead to skin damage, from premature ageing to an increased risk of skin cancer.

Beautiful, healthy skin is the result of a delicate balance between a nutritious diet and a healthy lifestyle. Understanding this interaction offers a proactive approach to cherishing, protecting and nourishing our skin from the inside out. After all, when we take care of our bodies, it shows through our skin.

Physical activity, stress and skin

The interaction between physical activity, stress and skin forms a complex tripod in the vast field of health and well-being. Exercise and stress management can have major effects on the skin, and here's how they are closely linked:

Physical activity: a breath of oxygen for the skin

Stimulation of Circulation: Exercise increases blood flow, which helps to nourish skin cells and maintain their vitality. This increased blood flow brings oxygen and essential nutrients to the skin while eliminating waste products, including free radicals.

- **Sweating**: Sweating eliminates impurities, which can help unclog pores and reduce acne. However, it's essential to wash after exercise to prevent sweat from building up and aggravating skin problems.
- **Stress reduction**: Exercise releases endorphins, often called "happy hormones". These molecules help to reduce stress, which can lessen its effects on the skin.

Stress: The Invisible Link with the Skin

- **Inflammatory reactions**: Prolonged stress leads to an increase in the production of cortisol and other hormones. These hormones can stimulate the sebaceous glands, leading to excessive sebum production and, consequently, acne.
- **Accelerated ageing**: Chronic stress can affect the skin's structure and hydration, leading to a loss of elasticity and the appearance of wrinkles.
- **Exacerbated conditions**: Stress can aggravate pre-existing skin conditions such as psoriasis, eczema and rosacea.
- **Immune repercussions**: Stress weakens the immune system, which can make the skin more susceptible to infection and slow down the healing process.

The Perfect Balance: Physical Activity Against Stress

Exercise is often seen as an anti-stress therapy. It not only offers aesthetic benefits but also plays a crucial role in regulating our body's response to stress. By incorporating a regular exercise routine, we can improve skin elasticity, increase radiance and, above all, reduce the damaging effects of stress on the skin.

The harmony between regular physical activity and effective stress management can be the key to maintaining healthy, radiant skin. Recognising this symbiosis and acting accordingly can lead to better skin health and improved overall well-being.

Integration of dermatology in a holistic approach to health

The holistic approach to health emphasises the integration of body, mind and spirit, recognising that all these elements are interconnected and affect a person's overall health. Dermatology, often seen as a speciality focused exclusively on skin conditions, fits perfectly into this holistic framework when considered in its entirety.

Body: The Visible Manifestations of Inner Health
> **Reflecting overall health**: Conditions such as yellowing of the skin can indicate liver problems, while skin rashes can be a sign of food allergies. The skin often acts as a barometer for the body's inner health.
> **Nutrition and skin**: Diet has a direct impact on skin health. Foods rich in antioxidants, omega-3s and vitamins can improve skin clarity and elasticity.
> **Toxins and excretion**: The skin plays a crucial role in the excretion of toxins. Recurring skin problems can signal an imbalance or accumulation of toxins in the body.

Spirit : The Psychological Impact of Skin Conditions
> **Self-esteem and body image**: Skin conditions, whether acne or psoriasis, can have a profound impact on self-esteem. The holistic approach recognises this interconnection and seeks to treat not only the disease but also its psychological consequences.
> **Stress and the skin**: Stress can trigger or exacerbate skin disorders. Holistic care assesses stress as a potential contributing factor and suggests ways of managing it.

Soul: Connection with Self and Environment
> **Wellness practices**: Techniques such as meditation, yoga or deep breathing can benefit the skin by

reducing stress, improving circulation and promoting better overall health.
- **Connecting with nature**: Using natural products, moderate exposure to the sun for vitamin D, and taking advantage of the benefits of nature (such as fresh air) are all essential for healthy skin.
- **Intuition and listening to the body**: The holistic approach encourages us to listen to our bodies. If something doesn't seem right for our skin, it's often the body signalling a deeper problem.

Dermatology, when integrated into a holistic perspective, offers a much deeper and more nuanced understanding of skin health. It doesn't just treat visible symptoms, but seeks to understand and treat the whole person, recognising that the skin is the outward reflection of our inner balance.

Chapter 24:
ALLERGIES AND SKIN TESTS

Fundamentals allergic skin tests

Allergy skin tests are diagnostic procedures designed to identify substances to which a person may be allergic. In dermatology, these tests are frequently used to diagnose allergies that manifest as skin symptoms, such as eczema, urticaria or contact dermatitis.

1. Why have an allergy skin test?
Allergic skin tests can help to :
    Determining the cause of an allergy.
    Prevent future reactions by identifying allergens and advising patients on how to avoid exposure.
    To guide treatment, such as the administration of immunotherapy (allergens in the form of vaccines).

2. Types of allergic skin tests :
    Prick test: A small amount of allergen is introduced into the skin using a fine needle. This is the most common method of testing for food, environmental and certain drug allergies.
    Patch test: Allergen-impregnated discs are placed on the skin for 48 hours. It is mainly used to diagnose contact allergies, such as those caused by perfumes, preservatives or metals.
    Intradermal test: A small quantity of allergen is injected under the surface of the skin. It is often used when prick tests are negative, but an allergy is still suspected.

3. Preparing for the test :
- Avoid taking antihistamines several days before the test, as they can distort the results.
- Inform the dermatologist of any medication you are taking.
- Avoid applying creams or lotions to the test area.

4. Interpretation of results :
After applying the allergen, the skin is observed for any reaction. An elevation of the skin, called a papule, surrounded by redness, generally indicates a positive reaction, i.e. that the person is allergic to the substance.

5. Advantages and limitations :
- **Advantages**: These tests are quick, generally inexpensive and can confirm a suspected allergy.
- **Limitations**: They can give false positives or false negatives. Certain factors, such as medication or active dermatitis, can affect the results.

6. Continuation of the test :
Once the allergens have been identified, the dermatologist will provide advice on how to avoid exposure to these substances. In some cases, immunotherapy may be recommended.

Allergy skin tests are a valuable tool for dermatologists to diagnose and treat allergies. Although these tests are not infallible, when carried out correctly they can provide invaluable information to guide patient management.

Interpreting and communication results

Diagnostic tests in dermatology, whether biopsies, allergy tests or simple skin examinations, require not only accurate interpretation, but also clear and empathetic communication of the results to patients. This process is essential to ensure optimal care, minimise anxiety and foster trust between patient and healthcare professional.

1. The importance of accurate interpretation:
   Basis of treatment: A correct interpretation is the first step towards an appropriate treatment plan.
   Avoiding medical errors: Misinterpretation can lead to unnecessary treatment or, worse still, neglect of a condition that needs immediate attention.
2. Preparing for communication:
   Anticipate questions: Patients are likely to have lots of questions. Preparing in advance means you can provide clear, comprehensive answers.
   Choosing the right time and place: It is essential to have a conversation in a setting where the patient feels safe and comfortable.
3. Communication of results:
   Be direct but empathetic: It's crucial to be honest and transparent while showing empathy, especially if the news is unexpected or worrying.
   Use simple language: Although the use of medical terms is natural for professionals, it can be a source of confusion for patients. It's best to simplify medical jargon as much as possible.
   Providing visual or written support: This can help patients to better understand their diagnosis and treatment.
   Active listening: It is important to allow patients to express their feelings and concerns and to ask questions.
4. Managing emotions:
   Recognising anxiety and fear: Even benign results can be a source of anxiety. It is important to recognise the patient's emotions and respond to them with compassion.

- **Offer additional support**: In cases where the diagnosis is particularly worrying, it may be useful to refer the patient to support groups or therapists.

5. Follow-up after communication:
    - **Plan the next step**: Whether it's treatment, another test or simple follow-up, make sure the patient knows what to do next.
    - **Reminders and resources**: Provide patients with written or online resources, as well as reminders for future appointments or tests.

Interpreting and communicating results is just as crucial as carrying out the tests themselves. Good communication strengthens the relationship between the patient and the nurse or doctor, ensuring better care and understanding on the part of the patient.

Care and monitoring allergic patients

Allergy is an exaggerated response of the immune system to generally harmless substances called allergens. Manifestations can range from a simple skin rash to a potentially fatal reaction such as anaphylactic shock. For the dermatology nurse, caring for these patients requires meticulous attention, in-depth education and regular monitoring.

1. Identification and diagnosis :
    - **Detailed history**: Understanding symptoms, their frequency, severity and potential triggers.
    - **Skin tests**: Carry out or refer to allergy tests to identify the allergens responsible.
    - **Working with allergists**: In complex cases, it is essential to work closely with specialists.

2. Patient education :
   Avoidance: Teaching patients how to avoid identified allergens, whether in their food, their environment or their healthcare products.
   Recognising symptoms: Helping patients to recognise the first signs of an allergic reaction.
   Emergency action plan: Draw up a clear and concise plan for the patient in the event of a severe reaction, including the use of an epinephrine auto-injector if necessary.
3. Treatment and intervention :
   Medication: Prescribe or recommend antihistamines, topical corticosteroids or other medications to treat or prevent symptoms.
   Long-term therapies: For severe or chronic allergies, treatments such as immunotherapy could be considered.
   Emergency management: Knowing how to treat an anaphylactic reaction and when to refer the patient for more specialist care.
4. Follow-up and adjustments :
   Regular assessments: Allergies can change over time. It is crucial to assess the patient's situation regularly to ensure that treatments are still appropriate.
   Medication re-evaluation: Ensuring that the medication prescribed remains effective and adjusting it if necessary.
5. Psychological support :
   Living with allergies: It can be stressful, especially if reactions can be severe. Offer emotional support and refer to support groups if necessary.
6. Promoting awareness :
   Raising public awareness: Allergies can be misunderstood. Educating the public, teachers and employers can help create a safer environment for allergy sufferers.

The management of allergy patients is complex, requiring a combination of medical expertise, education and support. With appropriate follow-up, however, these patients can live full and active lives, while effectively managing their symptoms.

Chapter 25:
DERMATOLOGY AND SEXUALITY

STIs and skin manifestations

Sexually transmitted infections (STIs) are infections caused by bacteria, viruses or parasites, spread mainly through unprotected sexual contact. While most of these infections target the genitals, many can also cause visible symptoms on the skin, underlining the importance of awareness and training for dermatology professionals.

1. Introduction :
   Nature and origin of STIs: From bacteria such as syphilis to viruses such as herpes, STIs cover a wide range of pathogens.
   Routes of transmission: Although sexual contact is the main route, some STIs can be transmitted by other means, such as sharing needles or skin-to-skin contact.
2. Common STIs and their skin manifestations :
   Genital herpes: Characterised by painful vesicles on or around the genitals which may burst, forming open sores.
   Syphilis: This bacterial disease progresses in several stages. Primary syphilis manifests itself as a painless chancre, usually on the genitals. Secondary syphilis can lead to skin eruptions, particularly on the palms and soles.
   HPV (Human Papillomavirus): Some types of HPV can cause genital warts, while other strains can cause warts on other parts of the body.
   Molluscum contagiosum: Causes fleshy papules with a smooth surface, often with a central depression, which can appear anywhere on the body.

3. Complications and co-infections :
- **HIV and skin manifestations** : People with HIV can experience a variety of skin symptoms, from herpes zoster to fungal infections, due to reduced immunity.
- **Co-existing STIs**: It is not uncommon for a person to contract several STIs at the same time, which can complicate diagnosis and treatment.

4. Diagnosis and management :
- **Tests and biopsies** : Accurate identification of the STI is crucial to effective treatment.
- **Topical and systemic treatments**: Depending on the STI, treatments can range from antivirals to antibiotics.

5. Prevention and education :
- **Protection and safe sex practices**: Using condoms and limiting the number of partners can reduce the risk of transmission.
- **Vaccination**: Vaccines are available for certain STIs, such as HPV.

STIs are not confined to the genitals and can have significant skin manifestations. An integrated approach, combining prevention, accurate diagnosis and appropriate treatment, is crucial to managing these infections and preventing their spread.

Education, prevention and advice

In dermatology, as in other medical fields, patient education and prevention are as crucial as diagnosis and treatment. By informing patients about appropriate skin care and offering them relevant advice, healthcare professionals can play a decisive role in reducing the incidence of skin disorders and improving patients' quality of life.

1. The importance of education in dermatology :
    Prevention is better than cure: Healthy skin starts with the right daily habits and an awareness of the factors that can cause or aggravate skin conditions.
    Patient empowerment: By understanding their condition and the steps they can take to manage it, patients are better equipped to make informed decisions about their skin health.
2. Education on basic skin care :
    Cleansing: Inform patients about the appropriate way to cleanse their skin, taking into account their skin type and specific concerns.
    Moisturising: Stressing the importance of regular moisturising and choosing products suited to their needs.
    Sun protection: Educate people about the importance of protection against UV rays, choosing the right sunscreen and applying it regularly.
3. Specific advice for various skin conditions :
    Acne: Advice on products to avoid, the importance of not popping pimples, and dietary habits that can influence the condition.
    Eczema and psoriasis: Focus on the importance of moisturising, avoiding triggers and managing stress.
    Skin ageing: Information on the effects of the sun, smoking and dehydration on premature skin ageing.
4. Prevention of skin diseases :
    Skin self-examination: Educate patients on how to regularly examine their skin for suspicious signs, such as changes in moles.
    Infection protection: advice on best practice for avoiding skin infections, such as regular hand washing and keeping wounds clean.
5. Management of chronic conditions :
    Educating patients about the chronic nature of certain skin conditions, helping them to understand the need

for regular monitoring and adapting treatment as required.

Education and prevention in dermatology are essential tools for ensuring healthy skin throughout life. By working closely with patients, healthcare professionals can not only treat existing skin conditions but also prevent new ones and improve patients' overall quality of life.

Tackling sexuality in dermatological consultations

In the world of dermatology, talking about sexuality may seem irrelevant to some, but it is an essential dimension of holistic patient care. Many skin conditions can have an impact on a patient's intimate life or be directly linked to sexuality, which is why open and respectful communication is so important.

1. Relevance of sexuality in dermatology :
    - **Skin conditions and self-esteem**: Visible skin conditions can affect self-confidence and self-esteem, leading to difficulties in intimate relationships.
    - **Sexually transmitted infections (STIs)**: Several STIs manifest themselves through cutaneous or mucosal symptoms.
    - **Side effects of medication**: Some dermatological treatments can affect libido or sexual function.
2. Creating a comfortable environment :
    - **Confidentiality**: Assuring the patient that everything discussed remains confidential, and complying with medical confidentiality standards.
    - **Non-judgement** : Approach the subject with neutrality, without prejudice or personal opinion.

3. Ask the right questions:
>   Instead of asking directly about sexuality, you can start the conversation with questions such as: "Does your condition affect your personal or intimate relationships?
>   When an STI is suspected, ask questions about recent sexual practices, partners and protection used.
4. Inform and educate :
>   If the patient has an STI, provide information on how it is transmitted, the precautions to be taken, and the importance of warning partners.
>   Educate patients about the potential sexual side-effects of prescribed drugs.
5. Working with other specialists :
>   If a patient presents with sexual problems linked to a dermatological condition, consider working with a sexologist, psychologist or other relevant specialists.
6. Respecting limits :
>   If a patient is uncomfortable talking about their sexuality, respect their limits and do not insist.

Sexuality is a fundamental aspect of the human experience, and is intrinsically linked to our physical and emotional well-being. In the field of dermatology, dealing with sexuality sensitively and competently is essential for comprehensive and effective patient care. Healthcare professionals must be equipped to discuss these issues in a respectful manner, while providing the necessary information and resources.

Chapter 26:
PATHOLOGIES NAILS AND HAIR

Recognition common ailments

The skin, the outer covering that envelops our body, is the mirror that reflects many internal processes. It is also the first line of defence against external aggression. As a result, it can present a wide range of symptoms, from slight imperfections to serious conditions. For the dermatology nurse, it is vital to recognise these conditions quickly and accurately.

1. Acne :
    Typically associated with puberty, acne can persist or appear in adulthood. Characterised by inflammation of the hair follicles, it manifests itself as comedones, pustules or nodules.
2. Eczema :
    Eczema, or atopic dermatitis, is a chronic inflammation of the skin that causes redness, intense itching and scaling. Its cause is multifactorial, combining genetic, environmental and immune factors.
3. Psoriasis :
    This chronic condition manifests itself as red patches topped with whitish scales. It can affect various parts of the body, including the scalp, nails and joints.
4. Herpes :
    Caused by a virus, herpes manifests itself as an eruption of small, painful blisters, often around the lips or on the genitals.
5. Warts :
    Caused by papillomaviruses, warts are benign growths that can appear anywhere on the body.

6. Urticaria :
> Hives are an itchy, red, raised allergic skin reaction, often triggered by medicines, foods or other irritants.

7. Fungal infections :
> Fungi can infect the skin, nails or scalp, causing itching, redness and sometimes oozing lesions.

8. Melanoma :
> This is an aggressive skin cancer, which often manifests itself as a change in the size, shape or colour of a mole.

9. Rosacea :
> This chronic condition is characterised by redness of the face, sometimes accompanied by small dilated vessels, pustules or nodules.

10. Couperose :
> It manifests itself as redness due to dilation of the small vessels in the face, particularly on the cheeks and nose.

Faced with the diversity of skin conditions, dermatology nurses must be vigilant and precise in their recognition. A rapid and correct diagnosis is essential to ensure effective treatment and improve patients' quality of life.

Interventions and specific nursing care

Nurses play a fundamental role in the field of dermatology. They don't just assist doctors; they also offer comprehensive care, advice, education and support to patients. Let's find out more about the specific interventions and care provided by these professionals.

1. Skin assessment :
> First and foremost, the nurse carries out a careful assessment of the patient's skin, noting the presence, location, size, shape and colour of any abnormalities

or lesions. This assessment is essential to determine the nature and severity of the condition.
2. Administration of medicines :
    Whether applying topicals, administering oral medication or injecting treatments, nurses must do so with precision and in accordance with the doctor's instructions.
3. Wound care :
    In the case of wounds, ulcers or burns, the nurse must clean, disinfect and dress the affected area, while monitoring for signs of infection or complications.
4. Patient education :
    A crucial aspect of management is teaching patients how to take care of their skin, how to use prescribed medication and how to recognise the signs of a worsening or complication.
5. Diagnostic samples :
    Nurses may take skin samples, such as biopsies or scratches, which are then analysed in the laboratory.
6. Phototherapy :
    For patients requiring phototherapy, the nurse prepares the patient, manages the equipment and ensures safety during the treatment.
7. Pain management :
    Many skin conditions can be painful. The nurse regularly assesses the patient's pain and administers the appropriate analgesics.
8. Psychological support :
    Skin conditions can have a significant impact on a patient's self-esteem and emotional well-being. The nurse offers support, listens and, if necessary, refers patients to specialists.
9. Post-intervention follow-up :
    After dermatological surgery or another procedure, the nurse monitors the patient, making sure that the wound is healing properly and managing any discomfort or complications.

10. Interprofessional collaboration :
    The nurse works closely with the dermatologist, but also with other health professionals (pharmacists, nutritionists, psychologists) to ensure holistic patient care.

The role of the dermatology nurse is vast and essential. Through their skills, expertise and compassion, they provide comprehensive, personalised care, guaranteeing patients the best possible treatment.

Practical advice for patients

As the body's largest organ, the skin requires special attention to maintain its health and radiance. Proper care of the skin and awareness of the various skin conditions can make a major contribution to prevention and rapid, effective treatment. Here is some practical advice for dermatology patients:

1. Adopt a daily routine:
Cleanse your skin with a gentle cleanser suited to your skin type. Moisturise daily and use sunscreen every day, even on cloudy days.

2. Keep an eye out for changes :
Monitor your skin regularly to detect any changes or the appearance of new lesions. Regular self-examination can help identify potential problems early on.

3. Avoid long exposure to the sun:
Protect yourself from the sun, especially between 10 a.m. and 4 p.m., when the rays are strongest. Wear a hat, sunglasses and protective clothing. Reapply sunscreen every two hours, and more frequently after swimming or sweating.

4. Eat a balanced diet:
A diet rich in vitamins, minerals and antioxidants contributes to healthy skin. Include fruit, vegetables, nuts and fish in your diet.

5. Stay hydrated:
Drink enough water throughout the day to keep your skin hydrated from the inside out.

6. Avoid smoking :
Smoking accelerates skin ageing, causes wrinkles and reduces blood circulation, making skin paler and less healthy.

7. Use suitable products:
Only use products that have been dermatologically tested and are suitable for your skin type. Avoid irritating or allergenic products.

8. If in doubt, consult :
If you notice any unusual changes, persistent itching, rashes or other skin problems, consult a dermatologist without delay.

9. Limit the use of hot water :
Showers or baths that are too hot can dry out the skin. Opt for lukewarm water and limit the length of your showers.

10. Avoid scratching:
If an area of your skin is itchy, avoid scratching. This can aggravate the condition and lead to infection.

11. Get informed:
Keep up to date with the latest skin care research and recommendations. This will help you make the best decisions for your skin.

12. Be patient:
Some skin treatments take time to show results. Be patient and follow your dermatologist's instructions.

Proactive, well-informed management of your skin's health can prevent many skin conditions and contribute to healthy, radiant skin. Following this advice and consulting a dermatology professional on a regular basis can help you maintain the health and beauty of your skin throughout your life.

Chapter 27:
NEW TREATMENTS AND THERAPIES

Exploring recent advances

Dermatology, like other medical fields, is undergoing constant progress thanks to research, technology and a better understanding of the biological mechanisms underlying skin disorders. Recent advances have revolutionised the way in which healthcare professionals treat skin conditions and offer new hope for patients. Here is an overview of some of the notable advances made in recent years:

1. Biological therapies :
These drugs, designed to target specific parts of the immune system, have transformed the treatment of conditions such as psoriasis and eczema. By targeting specific proteins that play a role in inflammation, these treatments can offer rapid relief with fewer side effects than traditional treatments.

2. Lasers and light-based technologies :
New-generation lasers can treat a variety of conditions, from birthmarks and wrinkles to tattoo healing. Treatments are increasingly precise, reducing recovery time and side effects.

3. Genetic diagnosis :
The ability to sequence DNA at an affordable cost now makes it possible to identify genetic predispositions to certain skin conditions, paving the way for more personalised treatments.

4. Skin microbiome :
Research into the role of bacteria and other microbes that live on the skin has revealed their importance in skin health. This understanding has led to the development of

products and treatments aimed at balancing these micro-organisms.

5. Targeted therapies for skin cancer :
Instead of relying solely on surgery, there are now drugs that specifically target the genetic mutations present in certain melanomas, offering patients another line of treatment.

6. Applications and telemedicine :
The rise of skin monitoring applications means that patients can monitor their skin conditions and communicate with their dermatologists remotely, which is particularly useful in remote areas or for patients with reduced mobility.

7. Gene editing technology :
Although still at an experimental stage for many dermatological applications, techniques such as CRISPR offer incredible potential for treating genetic skin diseases at source.

8. Nanotechnology :
Using nanoparticles to deliver drugs directly to target cells in the skin means that treatments can be administered more effectively, with potentially fewer side effects.

9. Stem cell therapy :
Current research is exploring how stem cells can be used to treat skin conditions ranging from wound healing to hair regrowth.

As technology and science advance, dermatology will continue to evolve, offering more effective, less invasive and more personalised solutions for patients worldwide. These advances, combined with better education and awareness, ensure a better quality of life for people suffering from skin conditions.

Gene and targeted therapies

The rapid development of molecular biology and genomics has given rise to a new era of therapies in medicine, and dermatology is no exception. Gene and targeted therapies offer immense hope for many patients suffering from skin disorders, particularly those of genetic origin or linked to specific molecular anomalies.

1. Gene therapy :
Gene therapy aims to introduce or correct genetic sequences into a patient's cells to treat a disease. In dermatology, the potential applications are vast:
- **Epidermolysis bullosa:** A genetic disorder in which the skin is extremely fragile and can become injured or blister at the slightest touch. Clinical trials are underway to use gene therapy to correct the mutations responsible.
- **Genetic hair diseases:** Specific mutations can cause hair loss or hair abnormalities. By targeting these mutations, it is possible to achieve hair regrowth or improve hair quality.

2. Targeted therapies :
Unlike gene therapy, which directly targets the patient's DNA or RNA, targeted therapies act on specific proteins or metabolic pathways involved in the disease.
- **Melanoma:** Specific mutations, such as the BRAF mutation, may be present in certain melanomas. BRAF inhibitors have been developed to specifically target these tumours, offering a better response in patients with this mutation.
- **Psoriasis:** Biological drugs such as anti-TNF or IL-17 inhibitors target specific cytokines involved in the inflammation of psoriasis, enabling remission of the disease in many patients.
- **Eczema (atopic dermatitis):** Drugs such as dupilumab act by inhibiting the IL-4 and IL-13

pathways, two key cytokines in the inflammation of eczema.

Non-melanoma skin tumours: Inhibitors of specific signalling pathways can target advanced or locally advanced basal cell carcinomas, offering an alternative or complement to surgery.

The future of dermatology looks bright thanks to these advances. The integration of molecular biology, genomics and personalised approaches will transform the way dermatologists treat their patients. However, these treatments require particular attention in terms of monitoring side effects, costs and accessibility for all patients.

The future of biotechnology in dermatology

The modern era of medicine has seen a growing interest in biotechnology, with revolutionary potential in many fields, including dermatology. These advances, combining biology, chemistry, genetics and technology, offer new perspectives for understanding, diagnosing and treating skin diseases. Here's a glimpse of what the future could hold for dermatology thanks to biotechnology:

Cell therapy: Beyond gene therapy, the ability to cultivate, modify and reintroduce cells into the body opens up new avenues of treatment. For example, keratinocytes or other skin cells could be grown in the laboratory, modified to correct a genetic anomaly and then grafted onto a patient.

3D printing of skin tissue: Using 3D printing to create personalised skin grafts could revolutionise the treatment of burns, chronic wounds and other skin conditions requiring tissue repair.

- **Nanotechnology:** Using nanoparticles to deliver drugs directly to target cells can improve the effectiveness of treatments while reducing side effects. Imagine creams or lotions containing nanoparticles designed to precisely target inflammatory cells in conditions such as psoriasis or eczema.
- **Skin biosensors:** Devices integrated into the skin itself could continuously monitor parameters such as hydration, pH or the presence of pathogenic bacteria, enabling early intervention before symptoms appear.
- **Personalised therapies:** By understanding the genetic and molecular profile of each patient, dermatologists could prescribe treatments specifically tailored to the individual, thereby increasing the chances of success.
- **Skin microbiome:** An increasing amount of research is focusing on the role of the skin microbiome, i.e. all the micro-organisms present on our skin, in health and disease. Biotechnology could help modulate this microbiome to treat or prevent certain conditions.
- **Augmented reality and artificial intelligence:** These technologies could help dermatologists diagnose skin disorders by superimposing images, information and analyses in real time during patient examinations.

The future of dermatology, with the contribution of biotechnology, is incredibly exciting. However, as with any innovation, it will be essential to ensure that these advances are safe, ethical and accessible to all patients. There will also be a need for ongoing training of healthcare professionals to ensure that they remain at the forefront of these developments and can offer the best possible care to their patients.

Chapter 28: HOSPITAL HYGIENE AND INFECTION PREVENTION

Importance of sterilisation and disinfection in dermatology

The skin is our first line of defence against external aggression, particularly infectious agents. When its integrity is compromised or when it is medically intervened upon, the risk of infection can increase. Dermatology, as a skin-focused speciality, often involves invasive procedures, from biopsies to surgery, laser treatments or injections. In this context, sterilisation and disinfection are crucial to ensure the safety of patients and healthcare professionals.

Infection prevention: Any procedure that pierces or compromises the skin barrier can introduce micro-organisms into the body. Proper disinfection and sterilisation of instruments reduces the risk of post-procedural infections, such as cellulitis, abscesses or more serious infections that can spread throughout the body.

Compliance with professional standards: Good medical practice includes adherence to strict protocols to ensure cleanliness and sterility. Failure to comply with these standards may have legal and ethical consequences for the practitioner.

Patient confidence: Patients must have confidence in the safety of dermatological procedures. Impeccable hygiene and visible sterilisation protocols reinforce this confidence.

Equipment longevity: As well as preventing infection, proper disinfection and sterilisation can extend the life of instruments and equipment, by preventing corrosion and other damage.

Protecting medical staff: Healthcare professionals are also at risk when treating patients. Sterilisation and disinfection also protect staff from potential contamination by infectious agents.

Preventing antibiotic resistance: By reducing the risk of infections, we limit the use of antibiotics, which helps to combat the development of resistant bacteria, a global public health problem.

Diversity of pathogens: The skin can harbour a variety of micro-organisms, some of which are resistant to common disinfectants. Adequate sterilisation and disinfection are essential to eliminate a wide range of pathogens.

Sterilisation and disinfection in dermatology are much more than just procedural steps. They are a fundamental part of medical practice, guaranteeing the safety, confidence and well-being of patients and professionals alike. In a speciality where the integrity of the skin barrier is often put to the test, these precautions are absolutely essential.

Risk management and prevention of nosocomial infections

Risk management and the prevention of nosocomial infections are key concerns for healthcare establishments. These infections, acquired during a stay in hospital or another healthcare institution, can have serious consequences for patients and generate significant costs for the healthcare system. Adopting a proactive approach to prevention is essential to ensuring patient safety.

Understanding the sources of infection: Hospital-acquired infections can be caused by a variety of pathogens, ranging from antibiotic-resistant bacteria to viruses. These micro-organisms can be transmitted by direct contact, by the hands of healthcare staff, through the air or by contaminated surfaces.

Hand hygiene: This is the most effective measure for preventing the transmission of infections. Staff must be trained and encouraged to wash their hands regularly and correctly, using soap and water or hydro-alcoholic solutions.

Cleaning protocols: Regular and thorough cleaning of premises, particularly high-risk areas such as operating theatres, is essential. Surfaces, instruments and equipment must be disinfected using appropriate agents.

Patient isolation: Patients who are carriers or suspected carriers of contagious micro-organisms must be isolated to prevent the spread of infection.

Staff training: Healthcare staff must receive regular training in good practice, infection prevention protocols and epidemic management.

Vaccination: Ensuring that staff and patients (where appropriate) are vaccinated against diseases such as influenza can reduce the risk of spreading infections.

Surveillance and audits: Setting up a surveillance system for nosocomial infections means that outbreaks can be detected quickly and action taken. Regular audits help to assess the effectiveness of the preventive measures put in place.

Management of medical devices: Invasive devices, such as catheters or respirators, must be handled with care and sterilised or replaced regularly to reduce the risk of infection.

Communication: Informing patients about the risks of infection, the symptoms to watch out for and the precautions to take can help them to play an active part in prevention.

- **Response to epidemics:** Having an epidemic response plan means you can act quickly to contain the spread and treat those affected.
- **Risk assessment:** Identifying high-risk areas, vulnerable populations and procedures likely to lead to infections is essential for targeting prevention efforts.

Preventing nosocomial infections requires a global approach, integrating training, monitoring, hygiene and the implementation of strict protocols. Everyone involved in the healthcare system, from doctors to patients, has a role to play in ensuring a safe environment and minimising the risk of infection.

The role of the nurse in implementing hygiene protocols

Nurses play a central role in preventing infections and ensuring patient safety in hospitals. Their training and their position on the front line of care make them key players in hygiene. Implementing hygiene protocols is therefore essential to their day-to-day practice. Here is an in-depth exploration of this crucial role:

- **Promoting hand hygiene:** Nurses are role models for the rest of the medical team, patients and visitors. They ensure that they wash their hands regularly and meticulously, while making those around them aware of this fundamental practice.
- **Use of personal protective equipment (PPE):** Nurses know when and how to use PPE correctly, such as gloves, masks, gowns and protective glasses. They also ensure that this equipment is

accessible and used by other members of the care team.

Training and education: Nurses take an active part in ongoing training on hospital hygiene, keeping abreast of the latest recommendations. They may also be responsible for training new staff in established hygiene protocols.

Monitoring and surveillance: As a central link in the patient pathway, nurses observe, report and manage any incidents or risks of infection. They often take part in hygiene audits and contribute to the collection of data on nosocomial infections.

Waste management: Nurses are responsible for the safe disposal of waste, particularly potentially infectious medical waste, by following strict sorting and disposal procedures.

Disinfection and sterilisation: Nurses ensure that the equipment used is properly cleaned, disinfected or sterilised, as required. They may also be responsible for regularly checking the effectiveness of autoclaves and other sterilisation equipment.

Preventing infections associated with medical devices: The nurse ensures that catheters are inserted aseptically, and that they are maintained and removed under optimum hygiene conditions.

Awareness and communication: It informs patients and their families about the importance of hygiene, gives them personalised advice and answers their questions, thereby reducing the risk of transmission.

Collaboration: Nurses work closely with hospital hygiene teams, helping to draw up, revise and apply hygiene protocols.

Responding to epidemics: In the event of an infectious outbreak, nurses are often on the front line in identifying cases, implementing barrier measures and taking part in crisis management.

Advocacy: Nurses can play an advocacy role within the institution for the allocation of sufficient resources to infection prevention, stressing the crucial importance of hygiene for patient safety.

Nurses are much more than simply executors of hygiene protocols. They play a major role in their implementation, dissemination and compliance. Their daily commitment guarantees not only the well-being of patients, but also the quality of care delivered within the establishment.

Chapter 29:
DERMATOLOGY AND AESTHETICS

The evolution of medical aesthetics

Over time, medical aesthetics has constantly been transformed, adapted and perfected to meet society's changing beauty aspirations, while incorporating technological and medical advances. Here's an overview of this exciting evolution:

Origins and historical development: Although aesthetic concerns have existed since antiquity, aesthetic medicine as a discipline really took off in the 20th century. Procedures such as rhinoplasty and breast reconstruction emerged in the aftermath of the two world wars, mainly to treat soldiers' wounds.

The 1980s and 1990s: With the emergence of liposuction in the 1980s, cosmetic surgery became increasingly popular. In the 1990s, the advent of Botox revolutionised non-invasive treatments, offering an alternative to surgery for wrinkles.

Technology and innovation: The 21st century has seen the advent of technologies such as lasers, radiofrequency, high-intensity focused ultrasound (HIFU) and cryolipolysis. These techniques have made it possible to treat various aesthetic problems without resorting to surgery.

Integration of a global approach: Beyond treating specific areas, the approach has become more holistic, seeking to improve the patient's overall appearance, not just an isolated feature.

Naturalness and prevention: While there was a time when medical aesthetics sought to achieve spectacular results, the current trend is to seek natural results, preferring 'prevention' to 'correction'.

- **Diversity and individualisation:** Recognition of the diversity of beauty standards and the need for individualised approaches have led to treatment protocols that are better adapted to each patient, taking into account their specific ethnic, cultural and individual characteristics.
- **Greater accessibility:** With the democratisation of aesthetic procedures, a larger proportion of the population has access to them. Lunchtime procedures", quick treatments carried out during the lunch break, have become popular.
- **Regulation and ethics:** Given the rapid growth of the sector, regulation has been stepped up to ensure patient safety and maintain high professional standards.
- **Trend towards non-invasiveness:** Non-invasive procedures, which do not require surgery, have gained in popularity thanks to their shorter recovery times and reduced risks.
- **The future: As** research continues, medical aesthetics could well incorporate advances such as regenerative medicine, gene treatments and the personalisation of treatments thanks to artificial intelligence.

Medical aesthetics has come a long way since its beginnings. While remaining true to its fundamental mission of improving appearance and self-confidence, it has adapted to new technologies, society's changing aspirations and ethical imperatives, while always ensuring the safety and well-being of patients.

Ethical implications aesthetics in dermatology

Aesthetics in dermatology, like other areas of aesthetic medicine, is marked by a series of ethical concerns. These ethical implications arise from the interaction between the desire to improve physical appearance, patients' expectations, doctors' professional responsibilities and the limits of medical intervention.

Societal beauty standards: The media and popular culture often impose strict beauty standards, influencing people's perception of 'beauty'. Should practitioners adhere to these standards when providing aesthetic care, or should they adopt a more neutral, patient-centred approach?

Informed consent: It is imperative that patients fully understand the risks, benefits, alternatives and costs of aesthetic procedures. This requires transparent and honest communication from dermatologists.

Commercialisation and conflicts of interest: Given that many aesthetic procedures are paid for directly by patients (without insurance cover), there is a risk that clinical decisions will be influenced by financial considerations rather than the patient's best interests.

Realistic expectations: Some patients may have unrealistic expectations about the results of cosmetic procedures. It is the dermatologist's responsibility to manage these expectations and avoid performing procedures that may not be beneficial or may even harm the patient.

Access and equity: As most cosmetic procedures are expensive, this raises concerns about equity of access to care, potentially reinforcing socio-economic inequalities.

- **Safety and competence:** With the rapid growth in demand for aesthetic treatments, many practitioners with no specialist training are able to offer their services. This raises ethical questions about the competence and quality of the care provided.
- **Treatment of minors:** Should cosmetic procedures be authorised for minors? If so, under what circumstances and with what precautions?
- **Psychological pressures:** Some patients may seek aesthetic solutions for problems that are actually psychological or emotional. Identifying and addressing these underlying problems is crucial.
- **Respect for patient autonomy :** To what extent should a patient's aesthetic desires be honoured, particularly when they appear to run counter to medical standard or clinical prudence?
- **Technological innovations:** New techniques and technologies are constantly emerging. Their early adoption, before their effectiveness and safety have been fully established, poses ethical dilemmas.

Aesthetic dermatology, while offering considerable benefits in terms of confidence and well-being, requires careful ethical reflection. Dermatologists must balance patients' wishes with professional standards, while navigating the complexities of modern medicine.

The role of the nurse in aesthetic procedures

The role of the nurse in aesthetic procedures has developed considerably in recent years. With the rapid growth of the aesthetic medicine industry, nurses play an essential role in ensuring quality, safe and patient-centred care. Here is an overview of the role of the nurse in this context:

Initial assessment: The nurse assesses the patient prior to any aesthetic procedure. This includes taking a medical history, assessing current medications and allergies, and understanding the patient's motivations and expectations regarding the planned procedure.

Patient education: The nurse provides detailed information about the procedure, its benefits, potential risks, post-procedural care and expected outcomes. This education ensures that the patient gives informed consent.

Preparing the patient: Prior to the procedure, the nurse may be responsible for preparing the patient, which may include cleaning the area to be treated, applying topical anaesthetics, and checking the necessary equipment.

Assistance during the procedure: The nurse often assists the dermatologist or cosmetic surgeon during the procedure, providing the necessary instruments, monitoring the patient and making sure that everything goes smoothly.

Post-procedural care: After the procedure, the nurse gives instructions on home care, monitors the patient for any adverse effects, and makes sure the patient is feeling well before leaving the clinic.

Follow-up: The nurse may be responsible for post-procedural follow-up, verifying healing, ensuring that the patient is satisfied with the results and addressing any complications or concerns.

Technical skills: In certain jurisdictions and under the supervision of a doctor, nurses can carry out certain aesthetic procedures, such as injections of Botox or dermal fillers.

Complication management : Nurses are often the first point of contact for patients who have concerns after a procedure. They must be trained to recognise complications and to know when to refer the patient to the doctor.

Continuing education: The field of aesthetic medicine is evolving rapidly, with new techniques, products and technologies. Nurses need to keep abreast of these developments and take part in ongoing training on a regular basis.

Ethical aspects: As mentioned above, aesthetic medicine has many ethical implications. Nurses must navigate sensitively, always putting the patient's needs and wishes first, while maintaining evidence-based practice.

Nurses play a versatile and essential role in the field of aesthetic medicine. From initial assessment to follow-up, they ensure that patients receive comprehensive, safe and high-quality care.

Chapter 30: CAREER DEVELOPMENT IN DERMATOLOGY

Specialisation opportunities

In dermatology, as in many medical disciplines, there are a range of opportunities for nurses to specialise. These specialisations enable professionals to acquire in-depth expertise in specific areas of dermatology, ensuring high-quality care tailored to patients' specific needs. Here are some specialisation opportunities for dermatology nurses:

Paediatric Dermatology: Specialising in the skin conditions of infants, children and adolescents. It covers conditions such as eczema, nevi, genetic disorders and more.

Cutaneous oncology: Focused on the prevention, detection, treatment and care of patients with skin cancers such as melanoma, basal cell carcinoma and squamous cell carcinoma.

Surgical dermatology: Focus on surgical techniques and procedures such as tumour excision, Mohs surgery and other corrective or cosmetic procedures.

Cosmetic dermatology: Focuses on non-invasive aesthetic procedures such as Botox injections, fillers, laser therapy and other anti-ageing treatments.

Infectious dermatology: Specialising in skin disorders caused by bacteria, viruses, fungi or parasites.

- **Immunodermatology:** Focuses on skin diseases linked to the immune system, such as lupus, psoriasis and pemphigus.
- **Photodermatology:** Focus on skin diseases linked to exposure to the sun and treatments using light, such as phototherapy.
- **Hair and scalp dermatology:** specialising in conditions such as alopecia, scalp infections and other hair-related disorders.
- **Wound care:** Focus on the management and treatment of chronic wounds, such as venous or diabetic ulcers and burns.
- **Genetic dermatology:** specialising in hereditary and genetic skin disorders.
- **Psycho-dermatology:** Focuses on the link between the mind and the skin, treating conditions such as psychogenic pruritus, trichotillomania, and other conditions where psychological factors play a key role.
- **Ethnic skin dermatology:** Focus on the particularities and skin conditions most common in certain ethnic populations.

The training required for these specialisations may vary depending on the region or country. It may include a combination of clinical training, theoretical courses and continuing education. Specialisation not only improves the quality of care, but also offers rewarding career and leadership opportunities for nurses.

Continuing education and updating skills

Medicine is constantly evolving, and health professionals need to engage in ongoing training to keep abreast of the latest advances, techniques and clinical guidelines. In the field of dermatology, this requirement is just as imperative. Here's how continuing education and skills updating can be approached for a dermatology professional, in particular a specialist nurse:

Courses and workshops: Many institutes, universities and professional associations offer courses, workshops and seminars on specific subjects, enabling nurses to familiarise themselves with the latest techniques and trends.
Conferences and congresses: Attending national or international conferences gives you access to cutting-edge research and presentations by experts in the field, as well as the opportunity to network with other professionals.
Additional certifications: Certain specialities or techniques may require additional certification. Obtaining these certifications not only increases competence, but can also open the door to new professional opportunities.
Publications and professional journals: Subscribing to and reading specialist dermatology journals on a regular basis helps you to keep abreast of the latest research and advances in the field.
Online training: With the rise of digital technology, many courses and training are now available online, offering flexibility for learners.
Simulations and hands-on training: For invasive techniques or new procedures, mannequin simulations or virtual reality training can offer a risk-free way of practising and acquiring skills.
Discussion groups and forums: Joining online forums or discussion groups allows you to exchange experiences, challenges and solutions with other professionals in the same field.
Membership of professional associations: Membership of professional associations can provide

access to dermatology-specific resources, training and regular updates.

Feedback and supervision: Working under the supervision of a senior member of staff or getting regular feedback helps to drive continuous improvement.

Involvement in research: Participating in clinical studies, systematic reviews, or even conducting your own research can greatly contribute to your knowledge and skills.

Continuing education is crucial for any healthcare professional. For dermatology nurses, it not only guarantees optimal patient care, but also strengthens their professional credibility, ensures career progression and meets the ethical and deontological requirements of the profession.

The future of dermatology: new advances and technologies

Dermatology, like many other medical fields, is constantly evolving. Technological advances, biomedical research and scientific discoveries are all converging to shape the future of this speciality. Let's take a fluid look at the promising prospects for the future of dermatology:

At the heart of the modern medical revolution, dermatology is undergoing profound change. Digital technologies, molecular discoveries and new therapeutic modalities are transforming the way professionals diagnose, treat and monitor skin diseases.

Telemedicine, which has already begun to take root, will become even more prominent. Virtual consultations will become commonplace, facilitating access to care for those living in remote areas or with reduced mobility. Thanks to advanced algorithms and machine learning, **artificial intelligence** tools will assist dermatologists in diagnosing skin lesions, offering accuracy that is often superior to that of the human eye alone.

On the therapeutic front, the explosion in **biological therapies** is now targeting diseases such as psoriasis and eczema at a molecular level, offering personalised treatments based on the patient's genetics. These treatments, which are less invasive and more targeted, reduce side effects while improving efficacy.

Nanotechnology is also making inroads in the field of dermatology. Imagine nanoparticles designed to deliver drugs directly to a diseased cell or group of cells, maximising the therapeutic effect while minimising damage to healthy tissue.

Biotechnology is extending to skin regeneration. Laboratories are already cultivating skin in the laboratory for burn victims or people suffering from serious skin lesions. In the future, this technology could even make it possible to create customised skin for patients, with specific characteristics.

Wearables, or wearable technologies, such as smart patches, will monitor skin health in real time, alerting users and doctors to any suspicious changes. This could prove particularly useful for patients at high risk of melanoma or other skin cancers.
Cosmetic dermatology is not standing still either. Ever more precise lasers, biodegradable fillers and innovative anti-ageing treatments are being developed, promising natural, long-lasting results.

However, these advances, promising as they are, come with their own set of ethical, regulatory and training challenges. But one thing is certain: the future of dermatology looks bright, with the hope of ever more effective, personalised and less invasive solutions for patients.

Chapter 31:
CONCLUSION AND ADDITIONAL RESOURCES

Resources for further study his knowledge

If you would like to learn more about dermatology, here is a list of relevant resources, ranging from reference books and specialist journals to online platforms and professional associations:

1. Reference works :
    "Fitzpatrick's Dermatology in General Medicine - a classic work often cited as the "bible" of dermatology.
    "Dermatology: 2-Volume Set" by Jean L. Bolognia, Julie V. Schaffer, and Lorenzo Cerroni - another highly respected reference work.
2. Specialist journals :
    Journal of the American Academy of Dermatology (JAAD) - a flagship publication for the latest research in dermatology.
    British Journal of Dermatology - a renowned journal offering high-quality research.
    Dermatologic Clinics - focusing on current literature reviews and updates on specific topics.
3. Online resources :
    DermNet NZ - a comprehensive online resource offering images, descriptions and treatments for a multitude of skin conditions.
    Medscape Dermatology - offers articles, case studies and news related to dermatology.

4. Associations and Organisations :
    - **American Academy of Dermatology (AAD)** - offers a wealth of resources for professionals, from industry news to continuing education.
    - European Academy of Dermatology and Venereology (EADV) - an organisation for dermatologists in Europe.
    - **International League of Dermatological Societies (ILDS)** - focuses on international collaboration in dermatology.
5. Conferences and courses :
    - Events such as the *Dermatology World Congress* and the AAD annual meetings provide excellent opportunities for continuing education, networking and learning about the latest advances in the field.
6. Online educational platforms :
    - **Coursera** and **edX** - offer courses in dermatology, taught by renowned universities.
    - **Derm101** - a platform dedicated to dermatology training.
7. Forums and discussion groups :
    - Forums such as *DermTalk* allow dermatology professionals to discuss, ask questions and share information.

These resources are a good starting point, but it's essential to continue to seek out up-to-date information and attend regular continuing education courses to keep abreast of the latest advances in dermatology.

Expanding your knowledge of dermatology requires reliable, up-to-date resources. For French speakers, here is a list of relevant resources:

1. Reference works :
    - "Dermatology and sexually transmitted infections" by Jean-Claude Beani and Bernard Guillot - a comprehensive guide for health professionals.

"Précis de dermatologie" by Henri Adamski and Arnaud Bourdin - a book aimed at medical students, but also useful for practitioners.
2. Specialist journals :
   Annales de Dermatologie et de Vénéréologie - a leading publication in the French-speaking world for the latest research in dermatology.
   Revue Française de Dermatologie - offers scientific articles, clinical cases and news from the field.
3. Online resources :
   Dermato-Info - the Société Française de Dermatologie (SFD) website for the general public, packed with useful information.
   Fondation Dermatite Atopique - an information platform on atopic dermatitis.
4. Associations and Organisations :
   Société Française de Dermatologie (SFD) - offers a wide range of resources for professionals, from industry news to continuing education.
   Association Française d'Étude des Allergies (A.F.E.A) - focuses on skin allergies and their treatment.
5. Conferences and courses :
   The *Journée Dermatologique de Paris* and the *Journées Dermatologiques de Nice* are not-to-be-missed events for French-speaking dermatologists.
6. Online educational platforms :
   Université Médicale Virtuelle Francophone (UMVF) - offers free courses in dermatology.
   Medflixs - a video-based continuing medical education platform for healthcare professionals.
7. Forums and discussion groups :
   Specialist forums such as those run by the *SFD* or other professional associations provide a forum for professionals to discuss clinical cases or specific issues.

8. Training centres :
   - Many universities and schools in France offer training courses, university diplomas (DU) and inter-university diplomas (DIU) in dermatology. For example, Sorbonne University in Paris, Claude Bernard University in Lyon, and many others throughout France.

It's always essential to check information sources regularly, especially in a field as dynamic as dermatology, where new discoveries and techniques are constantly emerging.

Professional networks and associations

Professional networks and associations play a crucial role in training, informing, networking and defending the interests of dermatology professionals. For French speakers, here is a list of the main networks and associations in the field of dermatology:

- **Société Française de Dermatologie (SFD)**: This is the main organisation representing dermatologists in France. It organises conferences and continuing education courses, and publishes clinical guidelines.
- **Laser Group of the French Society of Dermatology**: This group brings together dermatologists interested in the use of lasers in dermatology. It offers training courses, exchanges on best practice and research into new technologies.
- **Association Française de Dermatologie Pédiatrique (AFDP)**: This association brings together dermatologists specialising in children's skin disorders.
- **French-speaking Dermatological Society of Sub-Saharan Africa (SODEFRASS)**: An association

designed to promote dermatology in the French-speaking countries of sub-Saharan Africa.

Réseau de Dermatologie Esthétique et Correctrice (RDEC): focuses on the aesthetic aspect of dermatology, providing a platform for exchanging information on the latest techniques and innovations.

Syndicat National des Dermatologues-Vénéréologues (SNDV): defends the professional interests of dermatologists in France, addressing issues such as regulation, pricing and relations with other players in the health sector.

EADV (European Academy of Dermatology and Venereology): Although not strictly French-speaking, this European academy is important for French and Belgian dermatologists wishing to connect to a wider network in Europe.

International Federation of Dermatological Societies (IFD): This worldwide organisation encourages collaboration between dermatological societies in different countries.

Forum des Dermatos Francophones (FDF): An online platform that allows French-speaking dermatologists to discuss various topics, share clinical cases and keep up to date with the latest news in the field.

Research groups: There are several research groups which focus on specific sub-specialities or problems, such as the SFD Psoriasis Research Group or the Infectious Dermatology Research Group.

It is recommended that dermatologists and professionals in the sector join or become members of at least one of these organisations in order to keep up to date, expand their professional network and contribute to the advancement of French-speaking dermatology.

Personal development and professional in dermatology

Personal and professional fulfilment is a goal that many healthcare professionals, including dermatologists, strive to achieve. In dermatology, this sense of fulfilment stems from a combination of intrinsic and extrinsic factors.

1. Direct Impact on Patients :
Dermatology offers the opportunity to improve patients' quality of life. For many, skin conditions can have a profound emotional impact, ranging from simple embarrassment to self-confidence issues or even depression. By helping to treat these conditions, a dermatologist can make a significant positive difference to patients' lives.

2. Diversity of cases :
Dermatology is a vast field with a variety of conditions ranging from common ailments such as acne or eczema to more complex cases such as autoimmune diseases or skin cancers. This diversity can be stimulating and provides an opportunity for constant learning and growth.

3. Work-Life Balance :
Unlike some other medical specialities, dermatology can often offer a better work-life balance. Life-threatening emergencies are rarer, allowing dermatologists to work more predictable hours.

4. Specialisation opportunities :
From dermatological surgery to cosmetic dermatology, from paedodermatology to dermato-allergology, there are many sub-specialities that allow dermatologists to follow their particular passions and interests.

5. Continuous innovation :
With advances in technology and research, dermatology is constantly evolving. This offers exciting opportunities to stay at the cutting edge of medicine and to adopt new techniques and treatments.

6. Multidisciplinary interactions :
As the skin is a reflection of internal health, dermatologists often work with other specialists, which enriches their professional experience.

7. Academic and research opportunities :
For those who are inclined, there are many opportunities in academia to teach, conduct research and contribute to medical literature.

8. Professional recognition :
Being an expert in a specific medical field offers professional recognition, whether among peers, within the community or internationally through conferences or publications.

However, like any profession, dermatology also has its challenges. Managing patient expectations, the pressure to keep up with rapid advances and managing the administrative and entrepreneurial aspects of a practice can be stressful. Nevertheless, with support, continuing education and a balanced perspective, dermatology can be an extremely rewarding and fulfilling career.

Made in the USA
Monee, IL
02 February 2024